VETERAN HORSE HERBAL

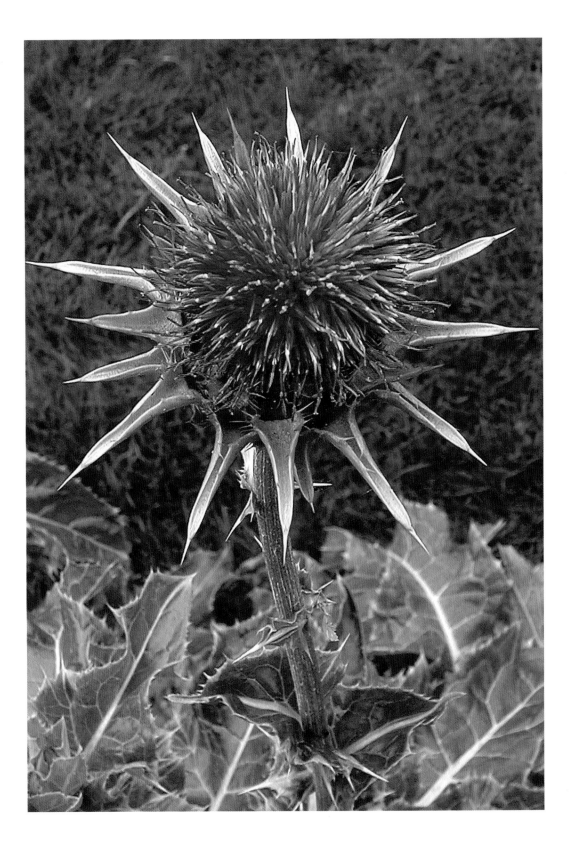

VETERAN HORSE HERBAL

Hilary Page Self
BSc MNIMH

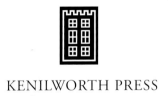

KENILWORTH PRESS

*This book is dedicated to Ditton (now sadly departed) and my
own horse Flamengo, two horses whose beauty 'fills the eye',
whose vigorous health confirmed my belief in herbal medicine,
and who have given me so much joy.*

❖

First published in 2005 by
Kenilworth Press Ltd
Addington
Buckingham MK18 2JR

British Library Cataloguing in Publication Data
A catalogue record for this book is available from the British Library

ISBN 1-872119-85-9

Design by Paul Saunders
Layout by Kenilworth Press
Printed in Singapore by KHL Printing Co Pte Ltd

Frontispiece photo: Milk thistle flower. (Photo by Annie Dent)

AUTHOR'S NOTE

All the information contained in this book stems from the author's
personal experience of using herbs on her own horses, and on those
belonging to other people, with veterinary supervision.

DISCLAIMER

This book is not to be used in place of veterinary care and expertise.
No responsibility can be accepted by the author, publishers or
distributors of this book for the application of any of the enclosed
information in practice.

Contents

❀

Acknowledgements 6

Foreword 7

Introduction 8

1 Herbal Preparations and Applications 11

2 Veteran Conditions and Ailments 24

3 Wounds and First Aid 74

4 The Older Horse's Diet, and Worming 79

5 The Veteran Competitor 85

6 The Final Chapter 89

Materia Medica 93

Glossary 96

Useful Addresses 98

Recommended Reading 100

Index 101

Acknowledgements

❁

This book was inspired by my husband's horse Ditton, who we sadly lost in 2001 at the age of twenty-nine. Ditton was a horse of a lifetime, a real gentleman; he taught Tony how to ride and my young horse how to behave! We are privileged to have known him.

Throughout his life, he was kept fit and healthy with the help of various herbal and homeopathic lotions and potions – we even named a couple of products in his honour. He also acted as a most patient and long-suffering model for many of the photographs in our advertising and catalogues.

For the last five years this book had been put to one side while I slogged away getting my medical herbalist's qualification. Thanks, Tony, for all your support, and for putting up with me during this difficult and exhausting period of my life. Never again, I promise!

My thanks also go to Julianne Aston of the Veteran Horse Society, who provided me with information and suggestions on which problems to cover in the book, for feedback on her Cushing's pony Timmy, and for the photograph of her fantastic veteran, Arthur.

To all the horse owners who so generously became involved in the Cushing's disease clinical trials I undertook as part of my final year's dissertation. This research would not have been possible without your help. I believe that the information gained through this trial will continue to help give many Cushing's horses and ponies a better quality of life.

In particular, I would like to thank Mrs E. Palmer of Bridport, Dorset, who very kindly agreed to let me use the photographs of her lovely pony Misty for the Cushing's section of this book.

To Dee and David Blunt at Kenilworth Press who were so supportive during my 'adult education' phase, and in particular to Lesley Gowers at Kenilworth who patiently prodded me to finish the manuscript (and only nagged me a little bit).

Finally, to veteran horses everywhere, who offer us unconditional love and friendship, and in doing so grace our lives with their presence – a truly rare experience.

HILARY PAGE SELF
BSc, MNIMH

Foreword

✿

WHEN DO WE CONSIDER a horse to be elderly? Many of us would say at around twelve years old, some a little older, perhaps at fifteen. What we do know for certain is that we have an ageing population of horses that are able to lead full and active lives well into their late twenties and early thirties, and often a fair way beyond that too.

This is in part due to advances in veterinary medicine, with better diagnostic techniques and therapies, coupled with a greater understanding of equine nutrition. It is also in no small way due to an increasing number of owners understanding the needs of the elderly horse and taking a direct and individual approach to their healthcare.

Ageing brings with it inevitable and inherent problems. The major organ systems gradually become less efficient, the senses less acute, the immune system weaker and the musculoskeletal system subject to degenerative changes and the effects of past wear and tear.

Fortunately, chronic conditions such as these respond well to complementary therapies. The same could be said of the majority of older horses, which benefit greatly from treatments of this type. Herbal medicine, homeopathy, flower remedies, nutritional supplements and a whole host of other treatments, coupled with sound, down to earth advice, can help alleviate many of the problems in a natural and supportive way often easing a condition where allopathic medicine has little to offer.

This unique book gives practical insight in using some of these therapies effectively to improve the quality of life and well-being of our veteran horse population. This will enable them to enjoy the later stages of their lives to the full, whilst at the same time, enriching the lives of their caring owners.

TIM COUZENS
BVetMed, MRCVS, VetMFHom, CertVetAc

Introduction

❁

Ageing is a natural process; however, few feral horses will achieve the advanced years that are reported by owners of domesticated animals. Natural predators, muscle weakness, degeneration of joints, or loss of teeth will ultimately lead to death, as a result of injury, starvation, or predation. It may seem to us that our horses have much the best deal in comparison with their wild counterparts. There are, however, pluses and minuses for the domesticated horse.

On the plus side is the provision of food, water, warmth, protection from elemental extremes and predation, veterinary care, farriery, dentistry, parasitic control, human ownership (not always a plus!) and care in old age.

On the minus side is the likelihood of increased exposure to unnatural environmental pressures and stresses, over-use of synthetic drugs and inoculations, conditions such as laminitis or digestive disorders through inappropriate diet or removal from natural habitat, development of joint problems as a result of repetitive movements, increased risk of parasitic burden through confinement in paddocks, inability to access the medicinal plants of 'nature's pharmacy', over-use of synthetic wormers, and the increased exposure to injury or even death in some competitive environments.

On the face of it, the odds would appear to favour the feral horse – but the fact is that there are not likely to be many forty-year-old feral horses; whereas domesticated horses, although exposed to the negative side of domestication, do benefit from the positive care they receive from their owners.

Caring for the ageing horse is not something that should be undertaken lightly. My experience has shown that if the job is to be done properly it can take as much, if not more time and effort than the management of younger horses in full work.

Domesticated horses have evolved to live and work closely with their human 'masters', and as such are totally reliant on their owners to provide for them. Unfortunately (as many welfare societies will confirm) it is often the case that the older horse whose owner feels he has reached the end of his 'useful' life will find himself discarded, turned away, and separated from the human companionship he has known all his life.

In the world of human resources businesses have identified the enormous contribution that the older generation can offer with their life and work experience. The veteran horse is no different, and is supremely suited to taking on the role of schoolmaster, providing a steadying influence, while helping to build confidence in young horses and novice riders. My own 'bomb-proof' veteran horse was a fantastic asset when our three-year-old youngster was first introduced to the busy roads around our property, inspiring confidence and setting an excellent example of how to behave in traffic.

In 2002 I was asked to give a talk at the UK's Equine Event, an annual show that attracts horse owners and enthusiasts from all over the country. On this occasion I decided to make the subject of my talk 'Keeping Your Veteran Viable Using Complementary Therapies'. I was overwhelmed with the response – the hall was packed to capacity and people were standing in the aisles!

What this so clearly illustrated to me was that not only are there a huge number of veteran horse owners, but that these owners are really enthusiastic about using natural therapies to help keep their veterans fit and well.

Ditton, at the age of twenty-seven. (Photo by Annie Dent)

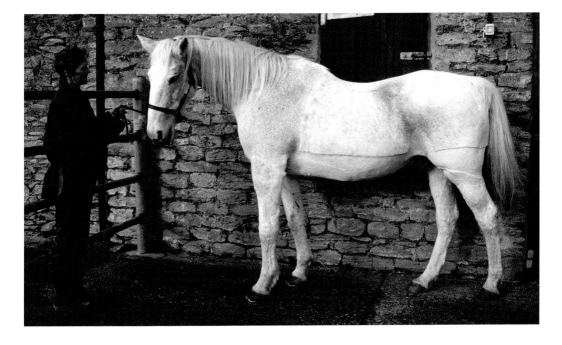

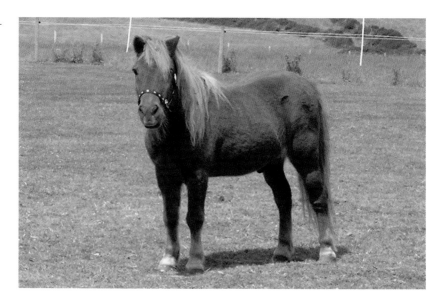

Arthur, a fifty-year-old Shetland pony belonging to the Veteran Horse Society.

On this same occasion I was introduced to the founder of the newly formed Veteran Horse Society (VHS), an organisation which I am pleased to say has since gone from strength to strength. The Society is now a registered charity with over 3000 members and is responsible for the welfare, rescue and rehoming of horses over the age of fifteen.

Each year the organisation runs a series of regional showing competitions, culminating in a championship class for the ten regional finalists, at Olympia in December. In 2003 over 2000 veteran horses entered the 468 qualifiers, with the Veteran Horse Supreme Championship being won by 'Hudson Bay', a stunning thirty-year-old Cleveland Bay x Thoroughbred ex-police horse.

In 2004 the Society succeeded in gaining 'Badger', a 14.2hh lovely grey Arab x Welsh gelding, a place in history, by having him included in the *Guinness Book of Records* at the age of fifty-one years!

To my mind, this not only shows just how many active veteran horses there are in the UK, but also goes to confirm my belief that with loving care and a bit of extra effort there is no reason why horses cannot remain fit and healthy well into their thirties and beyond.

Herbal and other complementary medicine is particularly suited to the older generation, be they people or animals. The medicine is gentle, can be administered in a variety of forms and is generally safe to use in conjunction with conventional medication. It is also particularly appropriate for the treatment of the more chronic conditions that tend to plague the older generation.

✿

CHAPTER ONE

Herbal Preparations and Applications

'Better to hunt in fields, for health unbought,
Than fee the doctor for nauseous draught'
JOHN DRYDEN 1631–1700

ONE OF THE MOST effective uses of herbal medicine is for the relief of long-term or chronic conditions that can persist in the elderly. Many of the problems they experience have developed throughout their lives and the gentle action of herbs can slowly but surely start to redress the balance and, in a time-honoured way, support the whole body, encouraging it to 'heal itself'.

If we assume that horses are like humans, then, in theory, the dosage of herbs, certainly those that come in tincture form, may be reduced for the older horse – body systems slow down and the active constituents of the plants take longer to be processed and excreted from the body. Certainly in allopathic medicine, dosages of drugs are reduced for the older patient, with quantities often dropping to those given to a child. In herbal medicine human patients over seventy would generally be given approximately three-quarters of the normal adult dose.

There are various ways in which herbs can be administered to the veteran horse and, depending on the condition you are treating, one method may be more preferable than another. There are now some really good books available that detail the collection, processing and production of various herbal remedies. If you are interested in growing and/or producing your own dried herbs, tinctures, creams, poultices, ointments and compresses, then I would suggest sourcing one of these books for in-depth instructions.

Here, though, is a brief overview on how herbs can be collected, dried and then used in the various preparations recommended in other parts of this book.

Fresh herbs/plants

Sourcing fresh health-giving plants and feeding them to your horse is the most natural and satisfying way of administering nature's pharmacy. Ensure that you collect them well away from busy roads or areas where chemical sprays have been used.

Probably the easiest way to feed fresh herbs is to let your horse choose them from local hedgerows, banks and ditches. Owners confirm that, given the option, their horses will ignore lush pasture and make a bee-line for plants such as hawthorn, couch grass, cleaver, oak leaves, meadowsweet, bay willow herb, beech leaves and cow parsley. This is not the horse being contrary, but rather it is acting instinctively to search out and eat plants it needs to maintain optimum health.

Fresh herbs are not only for internal use; many of them, such as comfrey, cleaver and mullein, for example, can be picked and used fresh to produce effective compresses.

Fresh herbs (roots, flowers, leaves, fruits and seeds) can be collected and fed to horses, dried for future use, or made into infusions, decoctions, oils, creams and tinctures. Aerial parts of plants and flowers contain large quantities of water, so you need to feed proportionately more fresh herb than dried herb.

If you collect fresh herbs for your horse, give him the option to accept or reject them. I gather a large bouquet of cleavers for our horses on most days during the growing season. I have found that they will eat it enthusiastically for several days in a row and then reject it. I take this to be the horse exercising its right to say no. At this point I usually give the horses a break for a few days and then try again.

It is worth remembering this fact if you are including a mixture of dried herbs in with the horse's daily food. Horses know what they need, and the only way they have of declining herbs that are combined with feed, is to refuse to eat! Should this situation arise, immediately stop adding the herb mix to the food. Once the horse starts eating again, add one herb at a time to the feed in order to identify which herb in the

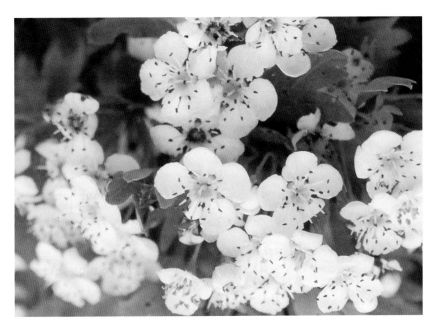

*Hawthorn.
(Photo: McOnegal
Botanical)*

mixture the horse is refusing. If using a commercially produced mix, contact the manufacturer. They should be happy to send you a small sample of each of the herbs included in their product so that you can test them on your horse.

Collecting your own plant material

Variations in plant material will occur depending on the time of day, season, weather, and type of soil – so bear in mind that this will affect the quality and quantity of plants available for collection. Picking the plants at the optimum time will ensure they contain the highest concentration of their active constituents.

Specialist books are now available that offer information and guidance as to the optimum time for collecting each plant. Always consult a good reference book to ensure that you are correctly identifying the plants you wish to harvest, especially if you are collecting them from the countryside. Only gather from healthy plants that show no signs of disease or insect damage. If you are picking plants like nettle or hawthorn, wear a pair of gloves to protect your hands, and always use a pair of scissors or a knife to avoid tearing or damaging the plant.

Harvest your herbs in dry, sunny weather after the dew has evaporated. Collect leaves as they open during the spring and summer. Pick flowers at, or just prior to, pollination. Berries and fruit are collected when they are fully grown and ripe. Seeds are collected in dry weather when they are fully mature. Roots and rhizomes should be collected in the autumn once the goodness has been drawn back into them from the plant above ground.

Drying your plant materials

Cut the whole stem with the leaf and/or flower heads attached. Strip the very bottom leaves from the stems, tie five or six stems together, and hang them upside down in a clean, dry, warm atmosphere where there is a good flow of air. This can be done in direct sunlight, providing the sunlight will not have any harmful effects on the plant's properties, otherwise hang in a barn, spare stable or airing cupboard.

Large flower heads such as calendula can be separated from the stems and laid on a tray on kitchen paper and allowed to dry. Once dry, the petals can be removed from the central stem.

Roots and rhizomes should be cleaned by first brushing the soil, debris and any pests away, and then washing in warm water. Chop them into small pieces or slices with a sharp knife and then spread the pieces onto absorbent kitchen paper on a tray. Place the tray in a warm oven that has been previously heated (and then turned off), for 2–3 hours with the door left slightly open. The warming oven of an Aga is perfect for this. Remove the tray from the oven and put in a warm place until the plant material is completely dry.

Flowers, leaves or roots can also be dried artificially, using trays that will allow a free flow of air. Employ temperatures of 40–60 °C for roots and 30–40 °C for leaves and flowers.

Herb storage

Correct storage of your herbal material is important. Once the leaves or flowers feel dry and slightly crisp to the touch, take them down and separate them from the stems by carefully rubbing the bunches over a large sheet of plain paper.

Place your herbs, flowers or roots in a suitable-size container such as a screw-top jar (preferably dark glass) or brown paper bag (do not use plastic). Make sure the containers are sealed well, then store them out of the light in a dry, cool atmosphere. Label and date the jars or bags, and try to use the herbs within about twelve months. Before using any of the material, check that it has not become mouldy or musty.

Commercial products

If you don't have access to fresh plants, or time to collect and dry them, then dried herbs are readily available. These can be bought either as commercially produced ready-made mixes or as individual herbs. Whichever form you decide on, it is vital to ensure that the quality is good, and that the company obtains the herbs from sustainable sources.

Herbs, like all foods, come in varying standards, from the weak and pathetic culinary herbs found in supermarkets to the robust wild herbs in our gardens and countryside. This equates, in food terms, to the difference between the factory farmed, intensively reared, artificially fed animal and the organically reared free-range animal with a natural diet.

Organically grown herbs are the ideal; however, they are expensive, not always available and beyond the pocket of most horse owners. Fortunately there is a happy medium, and there are still good supplies of herbs available that have been grown without the use of chemical sprays and from sustainable sources.

When you buy your dried herbs make sure they have a good colour and a nice fresh smell with no hint of mould or mustiness. Price is still a pretty good indication of quality, and you do tend to get what you pay for.

Plant sources

Unfortunately the indiscriminate harvesting of certain plants from the wild has led to deep concern among herbalists for the sustainability of some herbs. Many commercially available herbs and mixes are described as 'wild crafted' – to most people this conjures up a pleasing, healthy and wholesome image of wild herbs being carefully gathered in the countryside. Sadly, the reality is somewhat different, and in the past it has led to the destruction of wild habitats around the world and the loss of indigenous plant species

The trade in endangered plants is now an extremely profitable business, with plant species being added to the endangered list every day. When plants change hands for large sums of money there are plenty of individuals ready to take advantage and make a quick buck.

The herb golden-seal (*Hydrastis canadensis*) is one such plant. The plant's root stock is specific for any disorder of the mucous membranes, for fighting infection and for reducing inflammation. This plant has been harvested so indiscriminately in the wild (in North America) for both the domestic and international markets, that it is now endangered. Its whole-sale value has increased by over six hundred per cent in the last ten years and it has been placed on the CITES list (Convention on International Trade in Endangered Species). Thankfully, this fantastic plant is now being cultivated in both the USA and the UK, ensuring its beneficial actions will be available for generations to come.

The moral of this story is always to ascertain exactly where the herbs you buy are sourced from and whether that source is sustainable. As with the tea and coffee trade, there are now a number of Fair Trade organisations working to ensure that native people who grow and collect herbs in the third world, get a fair deal for their crops and are encouraged to replant for the future. For example, I buy my devil's claw from a supplier who sources this herb through an Oxfam-sponsored co-operative, to ensure the growers and workers in Africa get a fair day's pay for their work and harvest the crop in a sustainable way.

Using your herbs

So now that you have your dried herb, flowers, roots and seeds, what do you do with them?

The beauty of working with horses is that many of the herbs do not have to be cut or ground down to the size that would be necessary for human consumption. They can literally be added to the horse's daily feed, and most horses will find them extremely palatable. If, however, this is not appropriate, here are some other ideas on how you can produce herbal preparations for the elderly horse in your care.

INFUSIONS

An infusion is normally used if the active constituents of the herb are water-soluble. Infusions are particularly good for leaves and flowers, especially those that contain volatile oils, such as chamomile.

Making an infusion is just like making a pot of tea, and can be produced using one or a combination of herbs.

Take your fresh or dried herb and place it in a teapot or saucepan, pour in just-boiled water, replace the lid and leave to infuse for 5–10 minutes.

As a general rule-of-thumb, you should use approximately 20g of dried herb or 30g of fresh herb to 500ml of water.

Some herbs contain volatile or essential oils which will evaporate with the steam if the lid is left off. To prevent this happening ensure you replace the lid of the teapot or saucepan as soon as you have finished adding the water. I tend to use infusions for horses once the 'teas' have cooled, but if you are trying to reduce a fever then they could be given while still hot (not too hot, though).

Once prepared, your infusion can be added to food, syringed into the mouth, used to soak a compress, used as a wash or lotion, or added to a spray. The herbs that were used in the infusion should not be wasted and can be added to the horse's feed. Any left-over infusions can be put into a jam-jar or a jug with a lid and kept in the refrigerator for up to 24 hours. If storing herbal preparations in the fridge ensure that they have not started to ferment before using.

Decoctions

A decoction is used when the plant material being prepared is hard or woody, such as barks, roots, fruits or seeds, and using the infusion method would not be forceful enough to break down the tough exterior. As with an infusion, this method will only extract the water-soluble constituents contained in the plant.

As a general rule-of-thumb when making decoctions you should use 5 parts of plant material to 120 parts of water. So, for example, if you had 5g of dried burdock root you would add 120mls of water; or with 50g of dried burdock root you would add 1.2 litres of water.

Fresh herbs can also be used for making a decoction, but in this case you should double the quantity of herb material used, to allow for the water content.

Take your chopped-up plant material and place it in a saucepan that has a tight-fitting lid. Cover the plant material with the appropriate quantity of cold water and bring it slowly to the boil with the lid on. Lower the heat and then simmer gently for 15–20 minutes in order to extract as much as possible from the plant material. The liquid should reduce by approximately one third. Remove from the heat and allow to cool, then strain the liquid through a sieve, squeezing out any liquid from the plant material. Depending on what it is, I often feed the horse some of the cooked plant material.

Use the decoction in the same way as you would an infusion. Any spare decoction can be stored in a refrigerator for up to 48 hours. Always check before use that the liquid has not started to ferment.

Tinctures

These are generally made with a mixture of alcohol and water. The ratio between alcohol and water is determined by exactly which plant constituents you wish to extract. For example, a higher ratio of alcohol to water would be used if the constituents in the plant were non water-soluble (such as resins and oils), and vice versa. Tinctures are available in a variety of strengths (1:3, 1:4 and 1:5); they are stronger and more concentrated than infusions or decoctions and extract more of the plant's active constituents. Tinctures are readily available from herbal suppliers and good health-food shops.

The preparation and production of tinctures can be time-consuming, messy and requires a certain amount of special equipment. If you are interested in making your own tinctures or liquid extracts, I would suggest that you consult a good reference book to obtain detailed instructions. Tinctures are the most concentrated way of administering herbal medicine and are more quickly absorbed by the horse's digestive system than dried herbs. They can be poured onto the horse's feed or syringed directly into the mouth. As far as internal use is concerned, when it comes to horses I am a bit of a purist, preferring to mimic nature and give dried or fresh herbs whenever possible.

Some people are not keen on giving animals alcohol. This can be overcome by adding a small amount of almost boiling water to the tincture dose and leaving it to stand for 5 minutes, to allow the alcohol to evaporate. Once cooled, the mixture can be administered as normal.

Several tinctures can be combined, if necessary, although you should try to avoid mixing too many together. I normally try to keep it to five or six maximum.

Tinctures can also be used for topical application by adding them to a cream, lotion, wash, compress or poultice. The tincture disperses readily into water or a cream base and brings with it all the plant's beneficial actions.

Creams

The making of creams is beyond the scope of this book. However, a simple base cream can be easily purchased (such as calendula, or hypericum) and then selected tinctures, fixed or essential oils added to the base cream as necessary, depending on the application.

Washes or Sprays

These are easy to make yourself. An infusion of the appropriate herb can be prepared and used as a skin wash, spray or eyebath. Aloe vera gel or extract is now readily available from herbal suppliers or health-food shops and this can also be used as a base for sprays and washes. Depending on the application, tinctures and/or essential oils can be added to your infusion or aloe vera. Put the wash into an indoor-plant hand-spray, as this makes it much easier to access awkward areas.

Remember to shake the spray before each application in order to distribute the oil and plant tincture molecules evenly through the liquid. Keep any spare wash in the fridge for 24–48 hours and check that it has not fermented prior to use. I always have several aloe vera plants in the house for quick applications. Cut a section of leaf off the plant, split it lengthwise with a knife and then collect the gel by scraping the blunt edge of the knife along the inside of the leaf. Use the gel immediately; do not store.

Poultices

Poultices can be used to draw infection from wounds, ease sprains or reduce muscle and nerve pains, and they can be made from fresh, dried or powdered herbs. Some fresh plants can even be applied directly to the skin

Calendula flowers. (Photo: McOnegal Botanical)

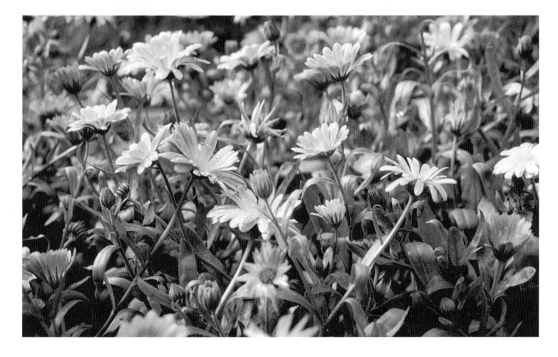

(midwives still recommend the use of bruised cabbage leaves, to help reduce inflammation in the breasts of nursing mothers). To use fresh or dried plants take enough herb to cover the affected area, place in a saucepan and add a small amount of water. Simmer for 2 minutes then squeeze out any excess water. Apply the herb while still hot (taking care that it is not too hot). Place a cotton pad over the herb and bandage in place.

For a poultice with a 'drawing' action for infections, wounds or thorns, use powdered slippery elm and powdered marshmallow root mixed with the appropriate tincture and warm or cold water. This mixture will produce a slimy paste that can be smeared onto a cotton pad and bandaged in place.

COMPRESSES

These are made from water-based herbal preparations such as infusions, decoctions and diluted tinctures. You will need about 500ml of your chosen infusion or decoction, or 25ml of tincture, added to 500ml of water. Soak a cotton pad or piece of towelling in the preparation and squeeze out excess liquid. Apply to the appropriate area and bandage over. Hot or cold compresses are particularly effective in helping to reduce swelling, bruising, inflammation and pain.

INHALERS

Essential oils can be absolutely invaluable for elderly horses, and inhalations using essential oils will relieve many respiratory conditions. I have found the following method to be a cheap and effective way of offering an inhalation to a horse. Line an old sacking nosebag, or one of those leather grazing buckets, with a cotton pad and then add a few drops of your chosen oil (e.g. tea tree, rosemary, eucalyptus, etc.) to the pad.

Place the nosebag on the horse so that the muzzle is a few inches away from the pad, and leave on for 5–10 minutes. The volatile molecules in the essential oil will be inhaled and carried to the limbic system of the brain and into the airways.

If applying essential oils externally, always dilute them in a carrier oil first as they may irritate the skin.

DOSAGES

This is not rocket science, and the dosage of herbs available to the public 'over the counter' is not as critical as for allopathic drugs. However, you do not want to give more herbs than are necessary, and some herbs are very dose-dependent, meaning that giving too much or too little can change their effect.

If possible, try to split the daily dose between two feeds. If, however you see your horse only once a day or have to rely on someone else to feed it, then the herbs can be added to one feed.

In general the following quantities would be given daily to a horse weighing approximately 500 kilos:

Tinctures: 15–20ml of a 1:3 tincture – if you are giving a mixture of several tinctures then give 15–20ml of the mixture.

Dried herbs: Approximately 30–40g

Fresh herbs: 80–100g. This will depend on the type of plant you are giving – for example, fresh couch grass root would be just a few grams, while fresh cleaver or nettle could be as much as 300g.

OTHER USEFUL THERAPIES

Bach Flower Remedies

I use this range of remedies extensively for both people and animals. There are 38 individual remedies plus the famous Rescue or Recovery Remedy. These remedies are made from flowers, shrubs, and trees and preserved in grape brandy. The flower remedies are designed to help with 'states of mind' more than physical conditions, although ultimately the state of the mind has an impact on the health of the physical body. There are now a number of really good books available which offer suggestions on their application for animals. The most important thing is to try to view the problem from the horse's perspective, and also be aware of how you, the owner, can affect the horse.

Storage – Bach Flower Remedies are supplied in 10ml dark glass bottles in a concentrated form, and have a very long shelf life if they are stored correctly. As with homeopathic remedies they should be stored away from electronic equipment such as microwaves, computers, mobile phones and televisions, and kept out of direct sunlight in a cool place.

Treatment and dosage – Flower remedies are normally given by mouth, with a course of treatment lasting approximately five days, although they can be given for longer. There are no side-effects. The flower remedies are absolutely safe and can be given in conjunction with herbal, homeopathic and conventional medicine. Depending on the situation, the remedy should be given at least three or four times a day, or more often if the condition is serious.

Having selected the appropriate remedy it can be administered in a number of ways:

- Drop 10 drops of the chosen remedy directly into the horse's mouth. This will only work if the horse is amenable and there is no risk of the glass dropper being broken or contaminated.

- Put 10 drops of the remedy onto a small piece of carrot, apple or a sugar cube.

- Add 10 drops to the horse's food. This method should only be used if you are confident the horse is 'eating up' and that the food is not going to be wasted.

- Add 10–15 drops of the remedy to every 4.5 litres (1 gallon) of the horse's drinking water.

- Add 10–15 drops of the remedy to water and use for topical applications.

Homeopathic Remedies

In this book I make reference to a number of homeopathic remedies that I have used on my own animals. I must stress that each animal is different, and consequently, the homeopathic remedy that is the most appropriate will vary depending on the animal's character, presenting symptoms, and case history. I suggest therefore that before using homeopathic remedies you consult either a homeopathic vet or one of the many excellent homeopathic reference books that are now available.

When I first started using homeopathic remedies on my animals the whole business seemed rather complicated and a bit daunting. It didn't take me long, though, to become much more confident, and I have had some fantastic results using homeopathic remedies on our sheep, cattle, horses, chickens and dogs. There are a few simple rules which I think are worth mentioning here.

- The remedies are an energy-based form of medicine, so they should not be stored near sources of electro-magnetic power, such as computers, mobile phones, microwaves, etc.

- Do not store the remedies close to strong-smelling products such as aromatherapy oils

- A dose is one pill or powder, or approximately 5–10 drops of a liquid remedy.

- The size of the animal is irrelevant – you give the same dose regardless of whether the patient is a mouse or an elephant!

- Try not to handle the remedies. The pills are coated on the outside with the remedy and if you handle them you will absorb some of the dose.

- Try to give the remedy into a clean mouth. The dose is given as soon as the tablet touches the mucous membrane.

- Do not add homeopathic remedies to the horse's food. Try to give the remedies at least 30 minutes away from food.

I find the easiest way to give homeopathic remedies to a horse is as follows:

- Take a small piece of apple or carrot and make a hole in it. Tip the tablet out of the remedy bottle and into the bottle lid, tip the tablet into the hole in the apple or carrot, and feed to the horse.

If you have an amenable horse then you can do the following:

- Take a piece of clean white paper and fold it in half, place the tablet inside the fold and close the paper, then crush the tablet using the back of a spoon. Pull down the horse's lip and tip the crushed tablet onto the inside of the lip.

✿

CHAPTER TWO

Veteran Conditions and Ailments

ALLERGIES

Including respiratory, dust, hay, seasonal and food allergies

RESPIRATORY, DUST AND HAY ALLERGIES

Recent years have seen a marked increase in the incidence of allergies experienced by horses, whether due to dust, hay spores, pollen or feed. In my opinion it suggests a lowering of the horse's ability to combat these allergens and a reduction in immune response, which may be due to environmental pressures, food or stress.

For the older horse, whose immunity may already be compromised, this is an additional concern. Prevention is always the better option, so if you know that your veteran has respiratory weakness or a propensity to allergies, you should try to strengthen the immune system and use herbs prophylactically prior to the danger period.

If dust or hay allergies are a problem then it may be worthwhile considering feeding haylage. This is now readily available in small bales, offers greater nutrition, is easier for the older horse to digest, is not dusty and is much better to handle than a soaking wet haynet! Admittedly haylage is more expensive than hay, but I have found that our older horses do better on it and retain more condition throughout the winter months.

Infection of the airways can occur more readily with the older more sedentary horse, who will find it harder to clear the lungs of mucus. Residual mucus in the lungs can create an ideal breeding ground for bacteria.

Thyme, **elecampane**, **garlic** and **plantain** are all excellent herbs, in that they will not only encourage the expulsion of residual mucus, but also have refrigerant, antibacterial and antiviral actions. If the horse has a temperature and cold/flu-like symptoms then use elder or boneset. These herbs will reduce fever and combine well with elecampane for respiratory infections.

Echinacea – this is the supreme herb for the immune system and can be used both prophylactically and curatively. In this instance it is specific for the upper respiratory tract and should always be given if there is danger of a spread of viral or bacterial infection (strangles etc.).

Liquorice – when used for the respiratory system this herb offers a mucilaginous action, relaxing the bronchials while also encouraging expulsion of mucus. Liquorice will soothe ticklish coughs and bronchospasm (as in asthmatic breathlessness).

I make up a thyme and liquorice syrup with elecampane and plantain tinctures. This is a fantastic cough syrup for those ticklish non-productive coughs that elderly horses so often have.

Seasonal Allergies

These are definitely on the increase with allergic rhinitis, hay fever, head-shaking, nose rubbing and sore, inflamed eyes as the most common symptoms. The principal allergens are grass and tree pollens, and crops such as oil-seed rape. In the end, however, horses are like humans, and can develop allergic reactions to just about everything! To help reduce the inflammation, irritation and allergic reactions use herbs such as:

Echinacea – this can help to strengthen immunity. It is specific for the upper respiratory tract, will reduce inflammation and has been clinically proven to help reduce allergic reactions. Just a note here: don't be tempted to cut costs by using the aerial parts of this plant. The roots contain the largest quantities of the active constituents, and, although more expensive, they are considerably more effective.

Chamomile – this plant has been found to be able to reduce the reaction to allergens such as pollen. Its anti-inflammatory action will soothe and heal the inflamed mucous membrane of the respiratory tract. In human herbal medicine it is used to help with anaphylactic shock.

Eyebright – this herb can be used both internally and externally. It is specific for allergies with mucus, and has a positive action on the upper respiratory tract, especially the sinuses. Eyebright has an anticatarrhal, antiseptic and anti-inflammatory action; it is astringent and will help to dry up watery mucus. An eyebath can be made to bathe sore, inflamed eyes. Certain cereals can encourage the production of mucus, so it is worth looking at your horse's diet if this is a problem.

Nettle – it may seem odd to use a plant like nettle for allergies, but it does have a very effective anti-allergenic action. It should be used for hay fever, asthmatic-type respiratory conditions, itchy skin, and insect bites. It combines particularly well with elderflower and can be given throughout the allergy period.

FOOD ALLERGIES

As with humans, food allergies in the animal population would also appear to be on the increase. A full investigation into the causes of this are beyond the scope of this book, should you have any concerns over your horse's diet then contact an equine nutritionist for advice. At the very least, the veteran horse should be provided with plenty of access to grazing, clean water, sun, fresh air, long fibre, not too much protein, and good wholesome food free from excessive sugars and processed cereals.

HANDY TIPS

Use a nose veil attached to the bridle noseband or headcollar to help filter the air and reduce the inhalation of irritating allergens. An old pair of tights provides a cheaper option, and works well for use in the field. Attach the mesh to the noseband of the horse's headcollar so that it hangs down over the nostrils.

Make enquiries about homeopathic remedies for allergic reactions to pollen – mixed pollen, mixed grasses, oil-seed rape. For allergic reactions to bites and stings, try Apis mel.

Bathe sore, tired eyes with an eyewash made from eyebright. Make an infusion of fresh or dried eyebright herb (see Chapter 1) and bathe the eyes three times a day.

APPETITE, LACK OF

As we get older our appetite tends to diminish in line with our reduced activity. Veteran horses are the same, but it is worrying when they 'go off' their food.

During the winter time this can be a real cause for concern for owners, who watch their sleek, rounded horse get steadily thinner and thinner. There is no replacement for 'Doctor Green Grass' and the majority of veterans will quickly regain the lost weight in the springtime, when the new grass appears.

I have already mentioned haylage under 'Allergies': I know that this is higher in protein than regular hay, but it is an excellent source of long fibre, is more readily digested, is softer and therefore easier to chew.

Be aware that worm damage, ulceration, stress, poor absorption of nutrients, inflammatory bowel conditions, scouring, Cushing's disease and tooth problems can all lead to weight loss. These are all conditions in their own right and are dealt with later in this book. In all of these situations, however, the horse would benefit from a probiotic, which should be used to help replace the beneficial gut bacteria. Weight loss can also be a sign of more serious conditions such as cancer, so always get your vet's opinion to rule this out.

Stress, separation from field mates, or stable vices can lead to a failure to thrive, lack of interest in food and subsequent weight loss. When we had to bring our twenty-nine-year-old in for longer periods during the winter, we stabled him in a large pen in our Dutch barn. This gave him lots of room to stretch his legs and keep his joints loose. He also had his best friend in an adjoining pen for company, and he had plenty of fresh air while being kept warm and protected from the elements. I appreciate that not everyone is lucky enough to have access to this sort of facility, but it is worth trying this arrangement if you do have a barn available.

In the past, the old pot-boiler was always the standby for keeping weight on horses during the winter. Barley and linseed would be simmered to produce an appetising mash, rich in oil and easily digestible. If you have the means to do this, then it is still worth considering, but for many horse owners this is too time-consuming and just not practical. Ready-steamed linseed is now available, and this provides an economical nutritious feed, rich in oil and vitamins, that will help to keep weight on, without heating up the horse.

There are several herbs that will help to put on weight or that can be used to tempt the shy feeder and encourage appetite.

Bitter herbs are good to help stimulate the appetite, although they should be avoided if ulceration is suspected. Bitters will increase the secretion of gastric juices, thereby stimulating appetite and improving the breakdown of food nutrients.

Herbs with bitter qualities include: fenugreek, artichoke, dandelion root, burdock, chamomile, yellow dock and mint. These herbs not only offer a bitter action but are helpful for a variety of digestive conditions. More of this later.

Fenugreek. This is better known as one of the ingredients in Indian cooking. The seeds can be sprouted just like bean sprouts; they are rich in oils, protein, calcium and vitamins A, B and C. Fenugreek is superb for poor digestion, especially in convalescence, and its oil and protein content make it a particularly nourishing herb.

Mint. It is no coincidence that commercial feed manufacturers include mint in their feeds, or that roast lamb is served with mint sauce! The plant stimulates appetite. It contains menthol, a volatile oil which increases production of gastric juices, soothes flatulence and nausea, calms smooth muscle cramping, and has a calming effect on the whole digestive system.

HANDY TIPS

Add apple juice, sliced apples and carrots to feed to tempt shy feeders. Grate the carrots to make them easier to chew.

Make feeds sloppy for elderly horses whose teeth are becoming worn. Do this by using very liquid sugar beet, or sugar-beet water.

Feed little and often. Remember: horses are grazing animals and prefer a steady trickle of food.

✿ Bach Flower Remedies

Gentian. This remedy is for lack of interest in food, especially if the horse will not eat when the food contains medication.

Arthritis

Including degenerative joint disease, ring bone, bone spavin, side bone, navicular, laminitis, muscle stiffness and rheumatism

I have included several conditions in this section because herbal medicine will generally approach the treatment of them in much the same way.

Depending on the nature of the problem, choose herbs from the list below, selecting those most suitable for the horse's condition.

As horses age they will ultimately suffer from a reduction in mobility, whether as a result of previous injuries, poor conformation, laminitis, hoof problems, degeneration of the joints, inflammatory changes, rheumatism, reduced circulation, muscle wastage, general stiffness or just wear and tear.

Herbal medicine takes a truly holistic approach to these conditions by using herbs whose actions will help to reduce the discomfort, address the cause of the problem, and then try to prevent any further deterioration. You should remember, though, that it can take years for some of these conditions to develop, so you must be patient and not expect instant results, although I have seen rapid improvement in many cases!

Select herbs that will help reduce pain and inflammation, cleanse blood toxins, assist in the excretion of inflammatory waste products, stimulate circulation and support joint flexion.

- **Anti-inflammatories and analgesics** to reduce the discomfort – devil's claw, meadowsweet, turmeric, yarrow, willow. Some herbs are most appropriate for specific areas of inflammation:

  Muscles and joints – devil's claw, meadowsweet, willow.

  Nerves – St John's wort. (I am always cautious when using this herb internally for horses, as there is a risk of prompting a photosensitive reaction in susceptible animals.) The oil can be used very effectively externally in any area where there are a large number of nerve endings.

  Eyes – eyebright.

  Bones – boneset.

- **Circulatory stimulants** – nettle, ginkgo, hawthorn, yarrow, prickly ash.

- **Vasodilators** – hawthorn, buckwheat, bilberry fruit, ginger.

- **Warming herbs** to improve blood supply to stiff muscles – ginger, turmeric, cayenne, rosemary, prickly ash.

- **Herbs whose constituents will neutralise** the acidic environment in joint capsules – meadowsweet, celery seed.

- **Depurative herbs** that will assist in the removal of waste products from the tissues – burdock, dandelion, prickly ash.

- **Lymphatic herbs** to support the lymphatic system in its role of cleansing impurities from the blood – cleavers, dandelion leaf.

Note: Non-steroidal anti-inflammatories (NSAIDs) are used extensively in conventional veterinary treatment for conditions such as laminitis, arthritis, etc. Many ponies and horses are given drugs such as phenylbutazone for weeks, if not months, at a time. It has been proven that these drugs can be detrimental to the digestive system, causing inflammation, oedema and ulceration. If you are giving NSAIDs to your horse I would suggest using herbs and a probiotic in conjunction with the drugs to help protect the digestive system and support liver function. See Chapter 4, on diet, for recommendations.

Boots, rugs and wraps containing static magnetic plates are now readily available; they can help improve blood supply to the extremities and large muscles masses. (Photos by Annie Dent)

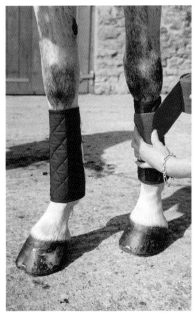
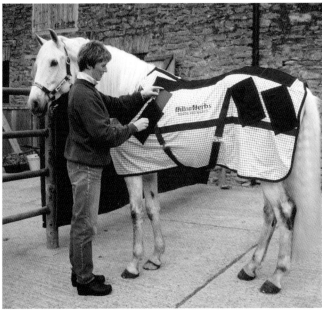

HANDY TIPS

Tackle these problems both internally and externally.

Bandage the legs of stabled elderly horses to help support the tendons, keep them warm and reduce the pooling of fluid in the legs.

Feed fresh cleavers whenever possible — they are diuretic, specific for the lymphatic system and can help to reduce filled legs and oedema. Good for laminitics.

Feed fresh nettles — cut them down and leave them to wilt for a few hours so they no longer sting. They are a fantastic circulatory stimulant as well as being rich in iron and vitamin C. Good for laminitics.

Massage areas of inflammation (joints or muscles) with lotions containing herbal tinctures such as arnica, ginger, comfrey or willow, and essential oils such as rosemary, lavender or peppermint. They can be easily absorbed through the skin to help shift lactic acid and toxic build-up, and the horse will really appreciate the massage. Be careful not to use too much and to dilute essential oils correctly.
A word of warning: These topical products can generate a lot of heat so if the horse has a sensitive skin do a patch test first; it is also not usually a good idea to bandage over the treated areas.

Give cider vinegar — this can be put into the drinking water or added to feed (50ml daily). The acidity of the vinegar will help to break down calcification and act as a blood cleanser. Try to source organic cider vinegar if possible.

Magnetic rugs and boots are now widely available and will improve circulation, which in turn will clear blood toxins from areas of inflammation and keep muscles warm and relaxed. Magnetic rugs, hock and fetlock boots, tendon wraps and pastern straps are all helpful for the older horse suffering from arthritis or rheumatism. Recent research undertaken in the USA has confirmed that magnets can increase blood supply, reduce pain, bring more oxygen to the tissues to promote healing, and carry away inflammatory bi-products such as histamines and prostaglandins.

❀ *Bach Flower Remedies*

Impatiens – if the horse is becoming irritable as a result of the pain.

Rock water – helps remedy rigidity and tightness; is ideal for arthritic pain.

Oak – for horses that have struggled with illness for a long time.

Beech – for tense, rigid horses that develop arthritic conditions as they get older.

Gorse – for laminitis, where the pain prevents the horse from resting.

❀ *Homeopathic Remedies*

Remedies such as Rhus tox, Ruta grav and Calc fluor/Heckla lava combination can be very effective for conditions such as arthritis, bone spavin, ring and side bone, splints, laminitis and navicular.

Each remedy is very specific depending on the presenting symptoms, so consult your homeopathic vet or a homeopathic reference book to identify which remedy would be most appropriate for your horse.

CANCER

This disease is beyond the scope of this book; and veterinary advice/treatment should always be sought. Depending, however, on the site of the cancer there may be herbs that can be used in conjunction with conventional medication. See the appropriate entry for herbal suggestions.

CUSHING'S DISEASE

In 2002 I undertook a clinical trial on horses with equine Cushing's disease (ECD) as part of my degree course in herbal medicine. I trialled the herb *Vitex agnus castus* on twenty-five ECD horses over a period of three months.

Not only was the trial encouraging, but it led to my gaining a far greater understanding of the condition, enabling me to consider other herbs to help and support the ECD animal. I must stress that the herbs suggested should not be considered as a cure; I have, however, had encouraging feedback from owners who report that they have helped. You can use conventional medication in conjunction with any of the herbs suggested here.

'Equine Cushing's disease results from adenomatous hypertrophy of the pars intermedia of the pituitary gland, which produces abnormally high levels of several hormones.' (Beech *et al*, 1985).

In other words, Cushing's disease is due to the development of a benign tumour of the pituitary gland. The growth of this tumour subsequently disturbs the delicate balance that normally exists between the pituitary gland, the hypothalamus, and the adrenal cortex of the animal, known as the 'negative feedback mechanism'. It is the disruption of this mechanism that leads to the presenting symptoms we all associate with ECD.

The hypothalamus is located in the brain stem and controls mechanisms in the body, such as temperature regulation, blood sugar levels, thirst, hunger, hormones and defence mechanisms such as the 'fight or flight' response. The hypothalamus interacts closely with the pituitary gland, which secretes the hormone ACTH. The release of this hormone into the bloodstream stimulates the adrenal cortex (located on top of the kidneys) to secrete glucocorticoid hormones (mainly cortisol).

These glucocorticoids have anti-insulin, anti-inflammatory and vaso-constrictive actions – it is this last action that can increase the risk of laminitis by restricting blood flow to the extremities. Corsitol, meanwhile, increases blood sugar by stimulating the liver to break down stored protein (gluconeogenesis).

In healthy animals, glucocorticoids are produced in response to stress: as the levels of these hormones in the bloodstream rise, they trigger an automatic feedback mechanism that 'instructs' the pituitary gland to stop producing ACTH (negative feedback mechanism). In the ECD horse this mechanism malfunctions and the pituitary gland continues to produce ACTH, which in turn prompts the adrenal cortex to release more gluco-corticoids. As you can see, this is a vicious circle and a self-perpetuating problem.

The increased levels of hormones in the bloodstream directly contribute to laminitis and are responsible for the diabetic symptoms shown in ECD horses such as:

- Weight loss
- Polydipsia – excessive thirst
- Polyuria – excessive urination
- Visual dysfunctions

ECD horses are also prone to repeated skin and organ infections. This is thought to be due to the cortisol, which depresses the horse's immune response, and the increased levels of blood sugar, which create an ideal environment for bacterial growth.

Cushing's disease is diagnosed by using the overnight 'dexamethasone suppression test' (the same test is used to diagnose Cushing's disease in humans). This test measures the amount of cortisol in the bloodstream, which is elevated in ECD horses due to the breakdown of the 'negative feedback system'. This test can be expensive to undertake and a large percentage of Cushing's horses are diagnosed simply on the strength of the number of presenting Cushingoid symptoms, such as:

- Hirsuitism – increased coat growth (often long and curly) with a failure to shed winter coat in spring
- Excessive thirst and urination
- Weight problems (increase or loss)
- Supra-orbital fat deposits – bulges over the eyes
- Fat pads
- Lethargy
- Depression
- Excessive sweating – hyperhydrosis
- Laminitis
- Spontaneous lactation
- Lowered immune response leading to recurrent organ and skin infections

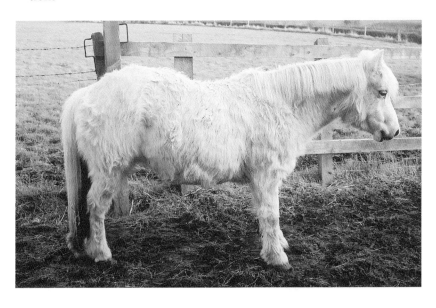

Misty, one of the ponies that took part in my clinical trial. This photo was taken just before the trial began, in May 2002, (Photo courtesy Mrs E. Palmer)

The conventional treatment for Cushing's disease is the drug Pergolide (a dopaminergic drug), which works by regulating the neurotransmitters dopamine and serotonin. Dopamine inhibits the production of ACTH by the pituitary gland.

Pergolide is not a cheap drug and it is important to establish the minimum dose required to control the ECD symptoms. Since the drug is a replacement therapy for dopamine in the pituitary, it must be given for the life of the horse. It is possible that the horse may become resistant to dopamine therapy, as is the case in human patients. For this reason the minimum dose is recommended in order to offset the risk of resistance developing.

That's got the scientific bit out of the way, now here's the herbal bit!

Why did I choose to trial *Vitex agnus castus* on ECD horses? I found details of clinical trials on humans that suggested the herb could have a similar (dopaminergic) action to the drug Pergolide on the pituitary gland.

With only twenty-five horses available, my trial was relatively small, but the results were encouraging and certainly warrant further research into the therapeutic effects of *Vitex agnus castus*. A significant number of owners on the trial reported the following improvements in their animals:

- Improvement in mood
- Reduction in hirsuitism (hairy coat) with a subsequent reduction in hyperhydrosis

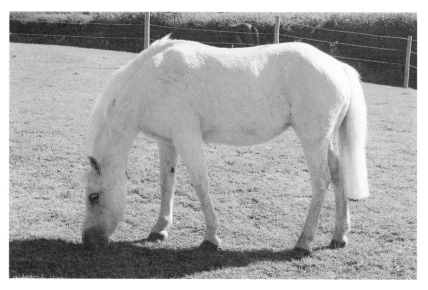

Misty, at the end of the three-month trial. (Photo courtesy Mrs E. Palmer)

- Improvement in energy levels
- Apparent reduction in the incidence of laminitis
- Reduction in the diabetic symptoms of polydipsia and polyuria.

In addition to the suggested herbs, it is important to remember that horses with Cushing's disease need an extremely high level of basic care and management:

- They will be more likely to suffer from recurrent infections.
- Wounds will be slower to heal due to their reduced immunity.
- Their feet will need extra attention because of the increased risk of laminitis.
- They will probably need clipping during the spring and summer.
- They may need to be clipped and then rugged up in the winter.
- If kept as part of a group of horses, their position in the herd may be challenged.
- Their diet will need special attention.

There are now a number of excellent websites which provide advice on feeding and managing the Cushingoid horse. I recommend reading an article written by the much-respected American veterinarian Joyce Harman, who is a keen advocator of herbal and natural therapies. The article was first published in the *Alternative Medicine Review,* September 2001, and the title of the paper is 'The role of nutritional therapy in the treatment of equine Cushing's syndrome and laminitis'.

As I mentioned earlier, my study of those twenty-five Cushingoid horses led to my gaining a far greater understanding of this disease. The following suggestions for herbs have been made because of their ability to help with the various aspects of the disease.

Vitex agnus castus – monk's pepper, chaste tree. The generic names for this herb originated as a result of their being used by young male novices in monasteries to help reduce their libido, and by women to help regulate their hormonal cycle.

In ECD animals the plant's dopaminergic action helps to reduce over-production of ACTH and other hormones that are linked to symptoms such as hirsuitism, spontaneous lactation, and depression.

Milk thistle – this is one of the most extensively researched herbs in human trials. Many vets are now using this in their practices for its ability to protect the liver from blood toxins and to speed up the renewal of liver cells. In Cushing's horses it will encourage the regeneration of liver cells

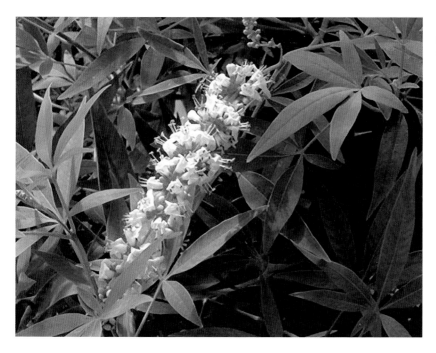

Vitex agnus castus. (Photo: McOnegal Botanical)

and protect the liver from the excessive corticosteroids in the bloodstream. Milk thistle is also an effective scavenger of free radicals with ten times the anti-oxidant action of vitamin E.

Golden rod – I am suggesting this herb because of its ability to support the microcapillary system of the kidneys, which are under extreme pressure due to the polydipsia and polyuria. Golden rod is also a very effective urinary antiseptic, and could help reduce the incidence of urinary infections that can occur due to the raised levels of glucose in the urine.

Artichoke – it is no coincidence that globe artichokes are eaten as a starter, at the beginning of a meal. They prepare the stomach for the arrival of food, encouraging the release and production of gastric juices. Use the bitter action of artichoke leaves first to stimulate gastric juices, and then increase the absorption of excess blood sugar and blood lipids.

Bilberry fruit – in the Second World War airforce pilots were given bilberry jam to help improve their night vision. Modern research has confirmed this action, as well as the fruit's ability to improve the micro-circulation of the eyes in people with diabetes and glaucoma. Cushing's horses suffer from increased pressure and damage to arterial and venous blood vessels in the eyes because of their diabetic condition. Bilberry fruit is not only an excellent wound healer but will also increase and improve blood supply to the extremities.

Goat's rue – Native ponies or horses that have evolved to live in very harsh conditions, such as Arabians and Welsh Mountain ponies, have been found to be insulin resistant. Insulin is the hormone that prompts cells in the body to absorb glucose from the bloodstream. Horses, like humans, can be resistant to the effects of insulin, leading to even higher levels of sugar circulating in the bloodstream. The herb goat's rue has been shown to reduce the absorption of glucose from the gut, increase the uptake of glucose by the cells and inhibit gluconeogenesis. Gluconeogenesis occurs in Cushing's horses when raised levels of cortisol in the bloodstream stimulate the liver to break down stored protein.

Echinacea – this herb should be used to help strengthen and support the horse's immune system, which is suppressed due to the excessive cortisol. Echinacea can be used on Cushing's horses internally to speed up the healing process of the body, and externally for wounds that are infected or slow to heal.

Hemp oil – I use this oil for myself, and all our animals. It is a plant source of the essential fatty acids Omega-3 and Omega-6. These fatty acids can help to make the cell walls more sensitive to insulin.

Note: Fish oils also contain Omega-3s but I prefer to use hemp (or flaxseed) oil for horses, as I am reluctant to feed 'animal' bi-products to herbivores.

MSM (Methyl sulfonyl methane) – this supplement is a source of bio-available sulphur. Sulphur is one of the components of the connective tissue found in the disulphide bonds of the laminae which connect to the hoof wall. Many Cushing's horses suffer from repeated attacks of laminitis so this supplement is worth considering.

Note: Cushing's horses are prone to repeated laminitis attacks and the conventional treatment for this aspect of the disease is the use of non-steroidal anti-inflammatories (NSAIDs) such as phenylbutazone, and circulatory stimulants such as isoxuprine. Chronic infection is another common symptom, often resulting in the use of high and repeated courses of antibiotics.

Many Cushing's ponies and horses are given these drugs for long periods of time. It has been shown that NSAIDs and long-term antibiotic use can be extremely detrimental to the digestive system. If you are giving these medications to your horse I would strongly advise using herbs that protect the lining of the digestive system and support liver function. I would also use a prebiotic and a probiotic after any course of antibiotics. See Chapter 4, on diet, for recommendations.

❁ Homeopathic Remedies

I have spoken to several owners of Cushing's horses who have successfully controlled the condition using homeopathic remedies, such as ACTH and Quercus robar. However, in view of the seriousness of this condition I would always recommend that you consult a homeopathic vet for advice on which is the most appropriate remedy to use.

❁ Bach Flower Remedies

Rescue/Recovery Remedy – this is for any occasion when there is stress or anxiety. Stress levels are high in animals with Cushing's disease.

Crab apple – this is a cleansing remedy which should be used for any sick animal as a detoxifier or whenever there is infection.

Gorse – this is the remedy to use when horses are ill, lacking in energy due to illness, have become lethargic or are suffering from painful conditions (such as laminitis) that prevent them from resting. Gorse should be used in conjunction with the flower remedy Gentian for horses with terminal conditions such as cancer.

Hornbeam – this is the remedy to use when there is cancer, or any condition which results in tiredness or weakness.

Oak – this remedy should be used whenever animals are weakened by chronic illness, fighting serious illnesses such as cancer, or are fighting to survive.

Olive – this remedy is for animals that suffer from long-term stressful illness, mental or physical exhaustion. This could be worth considering in view of the fact that Cushing's horses are in a constant state of heightened stress due to the hormonal imbalance.

Scleranthus – the keynote for this remedy is restoring stability and balance. It is a remedy used for helping with hormonal imbalance or illnesses that produce temperature fluctuations or changing symptoms.

DIGESTIVE DISORDERS

Colic, ulceration, irritable bowel, diarrhoea, scouring, constipation, and gut function, leaky gut, poor nutrient absorption.

As a horse ages, its digestive system will inevitably become less efficient. This can lead to scouring, dehydration, weight loss, bowel inflammation, allergies and many other conditions. A correct and healthy diet is vitally important, but this alone will not deal with any previous damage to the digestive system caused by drugs, stress, incorrect feeding, infection, parasitic burden, etc. Luckily there are many herbs that can really help improve the digestive environment, regulate gut motility, redress gut imbalances, reduce inflammation, improve the integrity of the intestinal tract, and support healing of gut lesions or ulceration.

Remember: the digestive tract starts in the mouth and ends at the anus. I will cover conditions of the mouth, teeth and dentistry under separate headings, but it is vital to ensure the horse's oral health and teeth are good if the horse is to get the most from its food.

COLIC

Colic is a life-threatening condition that is unpredictable and can rapidly become serious. If you think your horse is having a colic attack then veterinary attention should be sought as quickly as possible. The causes of colic are many, and include: compaction, trapped gas, parasites, overeating, stress, shock, ulceration and drugs.

If your horse is prone to colic attacks then there are herbs that you can use prophylactically to help reduce the incidence or severity of the attacks.

Valerian – most people think of this herb as a tranquilliser, but it is also a very effective antispasmodic. It will relax and reduce cramping of the smooth muscle in the gut. Use this herb if your horse is prone to spasmodic colic or stress-related colic attacks.

Cramp bark – as the name suggests, this herb will help relax smooth muscle and reduce cramping; it works particularly well in combination with valerian.

Chamomile – this is one of the best herbs for the digestive system. Chamomile contains volatile oils, it is anti-inflammatory, will reduce allergic reactions and is specific for gastro-intestinal spasm. Despite it having a sedative action on the nervous system, it is actually a tonic to the digestive system. It is effective against parasites and peptic ulceration, and can be used for food allergies.

Dandelion root – this is a gentle laxative, and can be used for mild indigestion.

Liquorice – this is the supreme herb for the digestive system – it is soothing to inflamed gastric mucosa and will increase production and excretion of gastric juices without altering the acidity. The Chinese have used liquorice for thousands of years in the treatment of gastric ulceration.

Gotu kola – this herb is currently being identified as another 'wonder herb', offering help in the treatment of cancer and HIV. Traditionally it is used to reduce scarring (internally and externally), as a venous tonic and as one of the principal healing herbs for both internal and external use. Studies have shown that it can heal and reduce the formation of peptic ulcers in humans and is useful for conditions such as Crohn's disease and ulcerative colitis.

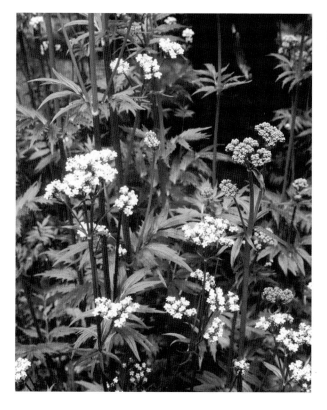

Valerian.
(Photo: McOnegal
Botanical)

HANDY TIP

Probiotics – gut flora and pH levels can easily become imbalanced particularly if strong purgatives such as castor oil have been used in cases of compaction. Use both prebiotics and a probiotic after treatment in order to help restore the natural gut flora.

✿ Bach Flower Remedies

Impatiens – this remedy is for any digestive problems such as irritable bowel, diarrhoea, indigestion and colic.

Recovery or Rescue Remedy – an all-purpose remedy to help with stress, tension and anxiety.

✿ Homeopathic Remedies

There are several remedies that can be given to the horse while you are waiting for the vet to arrive. The following are just a few recommended for digestive disorders, but you should consult your homeopathic vet to help you choose the right remedy, depending on the presenting symptoms.

• Colocynthus
• Nux vomica
• Carbo veg

ULCERATION

In the past, ulceration in horses was thought to be confined to the racing industry, but this is no longer the case. Foals as young as twenty weeks have been 'scoped and found to be suffering from ulceration.

Stress, lack of access to grazing and long fibre, drugs, bacterial infection, and high protein concentrate feed can all contribute to the development of ulcers. The horse fails to thrive, loses its appetite, becomes 'tucked up', is in pain, kicks at its belly, and may start to wind-suck or crib. In clinical trials, racehorses that had been diagnosed with ulceration improved once they were removed from the competitive environment and given access to grazing for just a few hours a day. If, therefore, the cause of the problem can be identified and removed, so much the better.

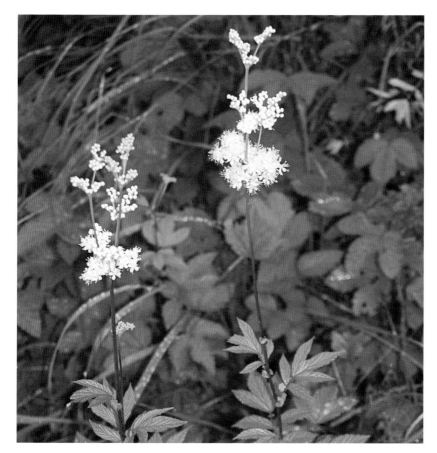

Meadowsweet.

Meadowsweet herb – is specific for ulceration; it can reduce acidity levels and inflammation in the stomach and encourage healing. It is an interesting fact that meadowsweet was one of the herbs from which an extraction was made to produce the drug aspirin (which we know can cause stomach bleeding). However, when the herb is used in its entirety it can actually heal and treat ulcers. This is a really good example of one of the principles of herbal medicine that 'the whole plant is greater than the sum of its constituent parts'. In recent years there has been a trend to identify and isolate the 'active' constituents in plants, which has led to the production of 'standardised extracts'. In general, these are an anathema to herbalists who know only too well the dangers of selecting a plant's constituents in isolation. The herb meadowsweet and the drug aspirin are a classic example of this.

Marshmallow root – this contains huge quantities of mucilage, a slimy constituent that can coat the surface of an ulcer and protect it from the acidic environment. If you want to see what this looks like, just soak a small amount of marshmallow root in cold water overnight!

Liquorice – this herb has been used for thousands of years in China for ulceration of the digestive tract. It is an effective anti-inflammatory, particularly for the stomach.

Comfrey leaf – also contains mucilage to help protect and encourage healing of the gastric mucosa.

Calendula – has the ability to increase the production of cells, both externally and internally. Clinical trials have confirmed its effectiveness in the treatment of gastric and duodenal ulcers. Calendula reduces inflammation and pain associated with ulceration and gastritis.

Slippery elm powder – valuable for ulceration and inflammation anywhere along the digestive tract. Like marshmallow it has the ability to protect the gastric mucosa from the erosive effects of acidity, and can reduce conditions such as diarrhoea caused by inflammation of the gut wall. Slippery elm is absolutely safe and can be used for the youngest foal or the oldest horse.

Gotu kola – specific for reducing inflammation in the digestive system, it can help with scarring both internally and externally and has been shown to be effective at healing ulceration.

DIGESTIVE DYSFUNCTION

Poor nutrient absorption, reduced gut efficiency, irritable or nervous bowel, leaky gut, scouring, constipation, gut damage, gut flora imbalance

All of these can be classed as digestive dysfunctions and will be helped by improving the integrity of the gastric mucosa. Food allergies, incorrect diet, stress and drug use, can all have a detrimental affect on the gut wall. In human studies the use of drugs such as non-steroidal anti-inflammatories (NSAIDs) has been linked to 'leaky gut' syndrome and to loss of integrity of the gut lining. In other human research the detrimental affect that antibiotics have on the gastric mucosa can still be seen two years after the course of antibiotics was given! Many veteran horses are given these drugs as a matter of course in the treatment of arthritis, laminitis or infections.

Poor integrity of gut mucosa and a breakdown in the basement membrane of the gut wall can allow large food protein particles to pass through and enter the bloodstream (leaky gut), setting up allergic reactions in the body. Inflammation of the colon and bowel can result in muscular spasm, cramping and scouring leading to weight loss and dehydration. Many skin and inflammatory joint conditions have been found to have their origins in digestive disorders.

Herbs should be used to improve the integrity of the gastric mucosa, reduce inflammation, encourage healing, and restore the balance of gut flora.

Most of us by now have heard of probiotics but more recently we are hearing of 'prebiotics'. These are dietary substances that favour the growth of the beneficial bacteria in the gut. They should be fed in conjunction with a probiotic to increase the production of beneficial gut bacteria, which will consequently improve absorption of food nutrients and digestion.

Note: For further information on prebiotics and probiotics see page 80.

Firstly use bitters such as yarrow, dandelion root, artichoke and wormwood to stimulate the appetite, increase gastric juices and aid digestion.

Choose herbs whose volatile oils will aid the digestion of food and reduce flatulence, such as fennel, peppermint, lovage and aniseed. Mint contains the volatile oil menthol, which produces light anaesthesia of the digestive mucous membrane. It will reduce cramping in the digestive tract and support liver function.

If you think there may be damage to the gut lining then use herbs such as: chamomile, marshmallow root, liquorice, gotu kola and slippery elm.

These herbs reduce inflammation and can repair and increase production of the cells that line the gut. This will speed up healing of gut lesions and ulceration caused by parasites, bacteria, drugs, or allergic reactions.

If the horse is prone to cramping or colic then select herbs that will have a relaxing and antispasmodic effect on the smooth muscle of the gut such as: valerian, chamomile, peppermint and cramp bark.

Elderly horses may be prone to developing bacterial infections, leading to the repeated use of antibiotics. I have found that a mix of 'antibiotic' herbs can be really effective. Garlic, thyme, myrrh, rosemary, lavender, calendula and peppermint all possess antibacterial and, in some cases, antiviral capabilities.

In a recent study carried out at the University of East London the constituent allicin that is found in garlic was shown to be effective against highly resistant strains of the notorious MRSA bacteria.

EYE PROBLEMS

As horses age, their eyesight will slowly deteriorate – just imagine how this must affect the horse both physically and mentally. The horse is an animal whose very existence relies on the 'flight' response to danger. Consider, therefore, how disadvantaged a horse must feel as its sight deteriorates or is lost. I have, however, known several horses who have lost the sight in one eye due to disease or accident who have continued to live a long and happy life, often pairing up with another horse to act as their look-out or 'second eye'.

Apart from medical conditions that affect the eyesight, poor diet, vitamin deficiency, parasites and allergens can all contribute to deterioration of the eyes. It is important therefore to ascertain the cause of the eye problem to help you select the appropriate remedy.

Eyebright – this herb has a special affinity for both the eyes and the sinuses. The herb is an antihistamine, is astringent, anti-inflammatory and anticatarrhal. Eyebright can be used internally for inflammation of the eyes, ears, mouth and throat, and externally as an eyebath. The plant is particularly effective for eye infections or irritation due to pollen or dust allergies. Like plantain it contains the constituent aucubin, which gives the plants their antiseptic action. I have used eyebright successfully to help both horses and dogs who suffer from corneal ulceration.

Bilberry is another extremely effective herb for visual problems. Clinical trials have confirmed that bilberry fruit can improve night vision (see also page 37), increase circulation and speed up healing in the micro-circulation of the retina. It is particularly good for individuals suffering from visual degeneration due to diabetes, and is one of the herbs I recommend for horses with Cushing's disease. Bilberry would certainly be worth using for any horse that has sustained an injury or blow to the eye.

Ginkgo – this herb is an excellent circulatory stimulant, being specific for improving the blood supply to the brain. In humans the herb has been found to improve blood supply to the retina and those parts of the brain that interpret the signals from the eyes, colour recognition and field of vision. In view of these findings I think it is worth considering for the older horse. In human herbal medicine, ginkgo is one of the principal herbs used for senile dementia.

Rosemary – this is one of the easiest herbs to grow; even those without a

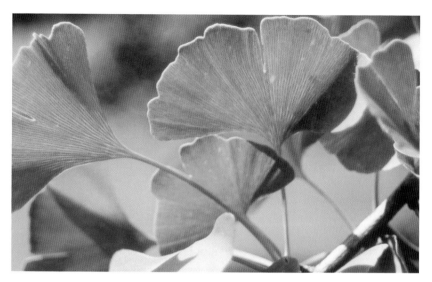

Ginkgo. (Photo: McOnegal Botanical)

garden can pick fresh rosemary all year round from a pot or window box. It contains a compound called rosmarinicin, which gives the plant its medicinal actions. Rosemary is particularly suited to the elderly, as it stimulates blood supply, particularly to the head.

HANDY TIPS

Eyebright eyebath – make a decoction by boiling 3g of the dried herb in 100ml of water for 2–5 minutes. Leave to cool, then strain the liquid and use to bathe the eyes at least three times a day.

Eyebaths can be made from a variety of herbs; the usual quantities are one teaspoon of the herb to one cup of boiling water. Make in exactly the same way as you would a cup of tea. Leave to cool, strain and then soak cotton-wool pads in the cooled tea and bathe the eyes. Ingredients for eyebaths, depending on the problem, are:

Infection – echinacea (make a decoction), clary sage, chamomile, plantain, elderflowers.

Allergies – eyebright, chamomile.

Inflammation – eyebright, fennel.

If you are in a hurry, or don't have any of the dried herbs, herbal teabags can be used – just soak in a little boiling water and then use the cooled teabag on the eye.

❁ *Homeopathic Remedies*

Euphrasia – this remedy can be used for conjunctivitis and other eye infections, including those with an allergic base. Use a few doses of arnica first for any injuries associated with the eye and surrounding area.

Moon blindness – this is a very distressing condition and you should always take veterinary advice on its treatment. There are several homeopathic remedies that can be used, such as Phosphorus 200c twice weekly to help prevent it worsening, Merc sol 30c once daily for soreness and ulceration, and Hepar sulph 30c twice daily if there is pus in the eye. As always, it would be wise to consult a homeopathic vet.

❁ *Bach Flower Remedies*

Elm – this is the flower remedy used to help with a feeling of inadequacy, and should be used for horses that are losing their sight, or hearing.

Larch – this is the remedy to use for lack of confidence. I think this remedy my be appropriate here, as any reduction in a horse's sight must have an impact on its confidence.

FOOT PROBLEMS

Corns, seedy toe, poor growth, poor circulation, thrush

'No foot, no horse' is an old saying, but a good one. It is important to remember that improving hoof quality and health is a long, slow process. Anything you feed will need to be given for at least six to twelve months before you can expect to see an improvement.

Most topical applications tend to be purely cosmetic, and in some cases can actually make the hoof more brittle. Don't be tempted to save money by reducing the frequency of your farrier's visits. Foot imbalance, corns and abscesses may remain undetected, causing discomfort and further problems if they are neglected.

Circulation in the older horse can be sluggish, and assimilation of vital nutrients, vitamins and minerals may well be reduced. This will inevitably impact on hoof quality and rate of growth. Previous laminitic attacks may have left the hoof wall weak and damaged; wet conditions and injury can also have an adverse affect on hoof quality.

Use herbs to stimulate circulation and improve blood supply to the tissues such as: ginkgo, bilberry fruit, nettle and alfalfa.

Herbs that are rich in vitamins and minerals which can improve horn quality include seaweed, cleavers and rosehips.

Tackle infections such as thrush by first cleaning the affected area with a strong salt solution, and then allowing the sole to dry completely. Apply highly astringent witch hazel, and then select essential oils made from plants known for their antifungal and antibacterial action, such as garlic, tea tree, calendula, myrrh and eucalyptus.

Mix your chosen oil/s with a carrier oil or gel and then paint onto the affected area. This treatment must obviously go hand in hand with the very best stable management if an improvement is to be achieved.

HANDY TIPS

When they are growing, pick cleavers and feed them to the horse – they are rich in silica (for strong hooves and coat) and will increase the production of white blood cells, thereby improving immunity.

There are homeopathic remedies that can help with poor hoof quality – check with a homeopathic vet for recommendations.

Use magnetic leg wraps or bell boots to help stimulate the circulation to the feet.

Use supplements such as MSM, a source of bio-available sulphur. Sulphur is one of the components of the connective tissue found in the disulphide bonds of the laminae, which connect to the hoof wall.

IMMUNITY, IMPAIRED, REDUCED OR WEAKENED

The immune system is a complex subject which cannot be regarded in isolation. Its effectiveness in protecting the body from disease relies on a variety of physiological systems working in harmony. Any imbalance in this harmony can contribute to a weakened immune response, or, in extreme situations, an auto-immune response. Diet, environment, disease, stress, pain and fear can all contribute to a breakdown in the body's natural response to disease or invasion by pathogens.

The veteran horse's immune system will naturally decline with age and is unlikely to be as strong as that of a younger horse. However, unless veterans continue to mix with horses outside their own environment, they are unlikely to be exposed to great risk of infection from disease. In addition, the older horse will have the benefit of a lifetime's immunity gained through exposure to, and resistance developed to, a variety of pathogens.

A healthy diet, attention to detail, prompt action when sickness occurs, along with extra care and attention will go a long way towards keeping your veteran horse strong and in the best condition to resist infection. There are herbs that can be used both to help strengthen the immune system and increase resistance to disease, as well as herbs that will help with infections should they occur.

Echinacea – this is the supreme herb for the immune system, and by now most people will not only have heard of the plant, but will also have taken it to help build up their own resistance to infection. A decoction of the root can be used topically to treat slow-healing wounds, bacterial infections or inflamed skin conditions. Without putting any additional strain on the immune system, echinacea can be used internally for weakened or suppressed immunity, and by supporting the body's immune response can increase resistance to infection. Echinacea has also been used to help reduce the allergic reactions that can lead to conditions such as head-shaking

Needless to say, there are many other herbs that can help the body fight infection and which one you choose will depend on the nature of the problem. The following herbs are all known for their ability to combat bacterial, viral or fungal infections.

Garlic – antibacterial, antifungal, antiviral, immune enhancing, antiparasitic.

Calendula – antibacterial, antiviral, antifungal.

Myrrh – antibacterial, antiviral.

Golden-seal – antiseptic, antimicrobial.

Thyme – antiseptic, antifungal, antiparasitic.

Elecampane – antibacterial, anthelmintic.

Plantain – antibiotic.

In addition to using herbs to combat infection, you should also select plants to strengthen and support the body, enabling it better to resist the disease state.

Herbs such as cleaver and couch grass will increase white blood cell production, thereby strengthening the immune response of the body.

Plants whose actions support liver and kidney function can help rid the body of poisons; these include milk thistle, cleaver, burdock and dandelion root and leaf.

Immunisation – in recent years, and particularly in the USA, research has suggested that changes should be made regarding vaccine protocols for cats and dogs. The recommendation is that the period between boosters should be changed from twelve months to three years. Research has also shown that the immunity conferred by these same vaccines can be as long as seven years, and may even be life-long!

I have to agree with the President of the Holistic Veterinary Medicine Association, Sue Armstrong, who stated that the practice of having to restart a vaccine schedule, even if the horse is only one day out of vaccine time, is outrageous, and that horses are grossly over-vaccinated.

The flu vaccine is also controversial, in that it may not even contain the same strain of flu virus as is currently prevalent. There is now a strong likelihood that competition horses competing under Jockey club or FEI rules will be required to be vaccinated against the flu virus every six

*Echinacea.
(Photo: McOnegal
Botanical)*

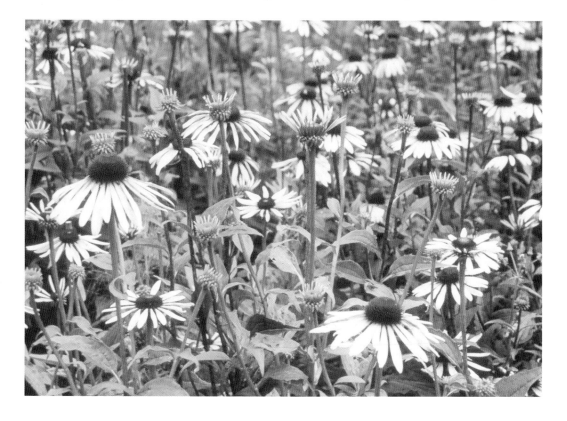

months! Would it be cynical to suggest that this could be just another attempt to boost the profits of drug companies?

Some drug companies have stated that side-effects and adverse reactions to vaccines are extremely rare. I would beg to differ: in the last three years, two of our horses have had adverse reactions to flu vaccines, and I have been told of five other similar reactions! I would suggest that adverse reactions are not as rare as the drug companies would have us think.

Last winter one of our horses was given his annual flu vaccine. It is a horse that we compete and we are therefore obliged to have him vaccinated. The horse was fit and well when he was vaccinated and in good health. This horse suffered from an adverse reaction to the injection, resulting in muscle stiffness in both the neck and quarters, and muscle loss. He took several months to recover fully. Our vet reported this to the drug company involved.

With regard to elderly horses, particularly those no longer competing, I believe that owners should weigh up all the available evidence, discuss the matter with their own vets, and then take a decision as to whether they wish to continue with the various annual boosters.

HANDY TIP

We are obliged to have conventional vaccinations for some of our horses and dogs because they compete or periodically have to go into kennels.

Prior to, on the day of, and for two days after our horses and dogs receive their conventional inoculations I give them the homeopathic remedy thuja. Our homeopathic vet advised us that this remedy helps the body prepare for and cope with the vaccinations. At the same time I also give a probiotic and milk thistle to support the digestive system and liver function.

Homeopathic vaccination nosodes are readily available from your homeopathic vet.

LAMENESS

The causes of lameness are many, and sometimes difficult to identify. I have covered several of these in other sections; however, I think it is worth mentioning a couple of other possible causes that may not be immediately obvious.

As horses age they generally continue to be ridden in the same saddle and bit that was used when they were younger, fitter, had better muscle tone, and probably better teeth.

Reduction in fitness, exercise or injury can very quickly result in the horse changing shape through loss of muscle tone or muscle wastage. This change of shape can radically alter the fit of the saddle, causing pinching of the nerves which enervate the muscles, leading to further wastage, possible discomfort and ultimately, the symptoms of lameness.

Rough or sharp teeth can also produce lameness symptoms. Pain or discomfort can cause the horse to alter the way it holds its head and neck, with the possible knock-on effect of spinal impingement, muscle stiffness, wastage and further problems in the neck or back. Make sure that as your horse ages you keep up those regular checks on tack and teeth to ensure your veteran stays comfortable in his work.

LAMINITIS – SEE ARTHRITIS

LIVER PROBLEMS

Liver function, protection, damage and regeneration

In the course of a horse's life the liver will come under tremendous pressure; it is vital that this organ be supported as much as possible if the horse is to continue to enjoy good health. The liver is responsible for bile production; carbohydrate, lipid and protein metabolism; conversion of glucose to glycogen for storage; maintaining and balancing blood glucose levels; detoxifying drugs and bacteria; processing hormones and worn-out red and white blood cells; storing vitamins and minerals; and many other functions without which the horse would quickly die.

Herbal medicine has always emphasised the importance of supporting the liver, and there are literally hundreds of herbs whose actions will ensure that it is kept healthy.

Bitters, such as dandelion root, milk thistle seed, artichoke, burdock and yarrow, will stimulate appetite and gastric juices and support liver function.

Protection of the liver cells from blood toxins is important. In clinical trials milk thistle seed has been proven to be able to protect the liver from

Milk thistle. (Photo by Annie Dent)

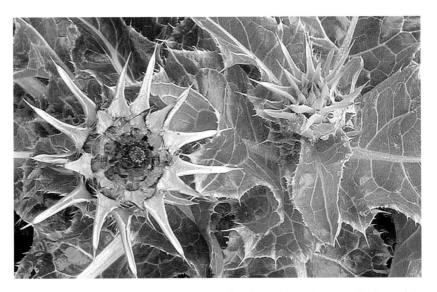

extreme poisons such as the amanita (death cap) mushroom. It does this by blocking the binding sites on the liver's surface membrane, thereby preventing uptake of the damaging toxins. Milk thistle has also been found to have ten times the anti-oxidant action of vitamin E, making it a highly effective free-radical scavenger.

The liver is one of the few organs that can regenerate and renew cells that have been damaged. The herb of choice for this action is also milk thistle, and, once again, clinical research has confirmed the plant's ability to increase the synthesis of RNA (ribonucleic acids), thereby supporting the liver's capability of regenerating new cells. Milk thistle is one of my favourite plants; I recommend it for use in conjunction with any medication or conventional wormer and for helping to repair liver damage. Milk thistle can also be used at the end of winter as part of a spring tonic, to help cleanse a sluggish system before the new grass comes through. It has been suggested that the herb is absorbed slowly by the body and therefore should be given for several weeks, if not months, at a time. I supply this herb to veterinary surgeons who have confirmed the herb's beneficial actions with liver enzyme tests.

Lymphatic System, Problems of

The lymphatic system is intrinsically linked with the bloodstream. Its principal action is to receive metabolic waste products from the blood. The lymph fluid containing these waste products is then filtered by the spleen and lymph nodes, sited in various areas of the body. Blockage of the lymphatic system caused by infection, trauma, injury, inflammation, tumour or swollen glands can lead to the development of swellings (lymphoedema) in areas such as the sheath, legs or jawline.

One of the most obvious signs of glandular activity can be seen in horses who develop an allergic reaction to something they have eaten in the field, and come in looking like a hamster! With swelling of the parotid gland, this condition, although unsightly, does not seem to cause the horse any discomfort and will usually resolve itself overnight if the horse is kept in. Some swellings, though, can be painful and may have further implications.

Many of the herbs that are good for the lymphatic system have antiseptic, antibacterial, anti-allergic and diuretic actions. This is particularly interesting when you know that disorders of the lymphatic system are usually due to the body becoming overwhelmed by infection, inflammation, enlarged glands or poor drainage.

Cleavers – another of my favourite herbs, is particularly effective for glandular swelling of the neck and 'armpits' of the horse. I like to use it in conjunction with its 'sister herb' calendula for all soft swellings, oedema and fluid retention. This combination is particularly effective for reducing filled legs and those hamster-like swellings. Mix the cleavers and calendula in an equal 50:50 combination.

Cleavers are diuretic and contain a constituent that increases the production of white blood cells; it will therefore also help with the immune system. Cleavers can be used externally as a compress for soft swellings, as can comfrey leaves.

Calendula – this plant has traditionally been used for inflamed or hard lymphatic nodes as well as for lymphadenoma. One of its constituents has been shown to have immunostimulatory properties.

Couch grass (the root) is used for glandular swellings. Horses and cattle eat the young shoots of the plant eagerly when they are first turned out after winter.

Seaweed (kelp, bladderwrack) is specific for the glandular system (thyroid gland in particular). It is rich in minerals and vitamins and contains large quantities of iodine.

Echinacea is a lymphatic and will strengthen immunity.

MELANOMAS

Melanomas develop as a result of the malignant proliferation of melanocytes (pigment cells). They are a particularly common occurrence in grey horses; they develop over a period of years and can cause problems as the horse ages.

My husband's horse 'Ditton' had melanomas when we bought him at the age of thirteen. We lost him at the age of twenty-nine, and during this time his melanomas grew steadily. He was fed a mixture of immune-enhancing, antimitotic and 'anti-cancer' herbs throughout his time with us, and I like to think that this helped slow the progress of the melanomas. These herbs included cleavers, burdock, echinacea, garlic and calendula.

The melanomas were particularly bad along the crest of his mane, around his anus and down his dock, and on occasions would burst open, oozing the dark black melanin (from which the melanomas get their name). When this happened I would bathe them with pre-boiled water to which I had added a few drops of hypericum and calendula tincture. Hypericum is specific for soothing sore and inflamed nerve endings, and calendula is antibacterial, anti-inflammatory and excellent for wound healing. I would then put on a soothing balm containing hypericum, garlic, propolis (antibiotic resin used by bees in their hives), honey (for healing) and calendula. As the melanomas grew around his anus, I made sure his diet included plenty of long fibre and grazing; this kept his droppings slightly soft, making them easier to pass.

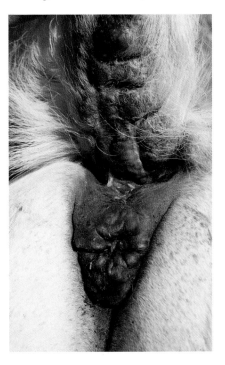

Melanomas around the dock and anus. (Photo by Annie Dent)

In more recent years my other grey horse's melanomas have started to grow larger. I have had success in reducing the size of one on his back by using a calendula base cream containing distilled witch hazel, which astringes and dries the area, and thuja tincture. Thuja is an antimitotic (inhibits cell division) –

antimitotics are used in human herbal medicine to help slow and reduce the division of cancerous cells. Antimitotics should not be applied to normal cells.

Another thing to consider when dealing with melanomas is the possibility of their development internally. During a rectal examination our vet found melanomas in Ditton's rectum. These would also break open periodically, causing inflammation of the bowel and diarrhoea.

❀ *Homeopathic Remedies*

There are homeopathic remedies, including nosodes made from melanomas, that are available. Contact your homeopathic vet for information on the appropriate remedy.

❀ *Bach Flower Remedies*

Crab apple – for internal cleansing.

Hornbeam –recommended for the day-to-day treatment of animals suffering from cancer.

MOUTH ULCERS

Older horses can be prone to mouth ulcers, and it is important to try to identify the causes of the problem. These can include lowered immunity; mouth/gum infections; sharp edges, points and hooks on teeth; food lodged around the gums; vitamin deficiency and poor diet. Mouth ulceration may also indicate more serious diseases, so it is important to rule these out. Cushing's disease can lead to a general reduction in immunity and mouth ulcers are one of the more common symptoms.

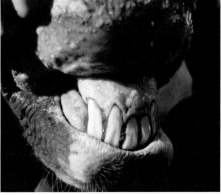

Ulcers on the gums.

Whatever the cause, the herbal approach to treatment will be the same. Firstly, help to heal the ulcers, and then address the underlying cause of the problem. Ensure the horse's diet is appropriate: it should contain plenty of access to grazing, fresh fruit and vegetables. Don't forget that vitamin B2 and vitamin C deficiencies can lead to mouth ulceration and poor gum health.

Horse with maxillary swelling. (Photo courtesy of R. Fisher BVetSc, MRCVS)

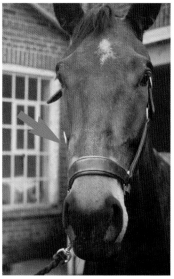

Poor dental hygiene is one of the biggest causes of mouth ulceration, so ask your equine dentist to check that the teeth are in good condition, that there are no loose, broken or sharp teeth and that the mouth is free from infection.

Abscesses in the mouth, or infected gums, can lead to ulceration, and in some cases the infection can spread up into the sinuses. I have known of several horses that suffered from repeated sinus infections and maxillary swelling, which would resolve with antibiotic treatment, only to return a few weeks later. The cause was later traced to the infected root of a tooth which had affected the surrounding jaw bone.

The following herbs will help to fight oral infection and encourage healing of ulcers.

Cleavers – feed fresh cleavers. The horse will love them. They are rich in silica, have a natural antibiotic action and are specific for mouth ulceration. An infusion of cleavers can be used as a mouth-wash.

Plantain or **mullein** leaves can be made into a tea and used as a mouthwash. They both contain mucilage, which will protect the ulcer and speed up healing.

Liquorice – anti-inflammatory and soothing, specific for both mouth and gastric ulceration.

Myrrh – this is a strong antiseptic as well as an anti-inflammatory. It can be added to any of the mouth-washes to help heal an ulcer and deal with any infection present. If the horse will allow it, myrrh tincture can be dropped or painted directly onto the ulcer(s), especially if on the lips. (This can tingle, so try a little of the tincture on your own lip first so you know what the horse is experiencing.)

Fresh garlic – feed four to five fresh garlic cloves daily. Most horses will eat them readily out of the hand. Garlic is antiseptic, antibacterial, anti-fungal, and a natural probiotic.

Sage – this can be made into a tea and then either syringed into the mouth or given as a very sloppy feed. Sage is antimicrobial, antiseptic, and specific for any oral inflammation.

Echinacea – this will increase the production of saliva in the mouth and provide an immune-enhancing and anti-inflammatory action.

Calendula – antiseptic, antifungal, healing and anti-inflammatory.

Chamomile – contains a volatile oil which is antimicrobial and anti-inflammatory.

If the horse is getting repeated sinus problems as a result of infection in the mouth then use **eyebright** herb internally.

MUCUS – SEE RESPIRATORY PROBLEMS

MUSCLE STIFFNESS – SEE ARTHRITIS

MUSCLE WASTAGE – ALSO SEE LAMENESS

Muscle wastage can be caused in a number of ways. In the older horse it can develop when exercise is reduced or discontinued, leading to lack of tone and muscle function. It can also develop if the horse is injured, and has to be confined to a stable. Muscle wastage can occur through lack of innervation of the muscle by the nervous system, as a result of pain, poorly fitting tack and skeletal injury.

RESPIRATORY PROBLEMS

Coughs, infections, mucus, sinuses

The respiratory system is a fantastic machine: it arranges for oxygen to be brought into the lungs via the bronchi and bronchioles and then to be exchanged for carbon dioxide in the alveoli. A healthy heart and good circulation have a direct involvement in this exchange of gases and it is important to remember that heart problems will inevitably lead to breathing difficulties and oedema.

The airways are protected from inflammation and infection by a lining of mucous membrane that contains a constantly moving escalator of tiny hairs (cilia). These hairs vibrate and help carry any irritants, allergens and excess mucus up and out of the horse's lungs and airways. The resulting reflex action of coughing is a protective measure that encourages expulsion of the irritant or mucus from the airways.

As horses age, this mechanism may become less efficient, leading to a build up of mucus in the lower airways, which can quickly become an ideal breeding ground for bacteria. As a result, infection flourishes, with its resulting inflammation, prompting the body to produce even more mucus, and so a vicious cycle develops.

This mucus can become tough and even harder to expel, the horse may develop a dry non-productive cough, the exchange of gases will be further hindered, circulation of oxygenated blood back to the heart will be reduced and the breathing can become shallow and laboured. In cases like this, veterinary help should always be sought.

Where allergies are concerned (these are dealt with on page 24), prevention is always better than cure, so take care wherever possible to protect the horse from exposure to allergens and infection. Generally, when the horse is out at grass he will have plenty of fresh air and be getting his head down, which will help to encourage the removal of mucus. As winter approaches, many older horses will spend part, if not all, of their day in a stable, where the air flow may be reduced and exposure to allergens or bacterial and viral infection is increased.

If you know that your horse is prone to hay/dust allergies, or has suffered with respiratory problems in the past, then start planning his stable management at least one month before he is due to be brought in. Ensure that the stable has a really good free flow of fresh air, and choose an appropriate bedding to further reduce any dust or spores. Select and start giving herbs to help support the respiratory system and reduce the risk of infection or allergic reactions.

Needless to say, it is important to keep the bedding clean and fresh, to further reduce dust or the risk of infection. A spray containing essential oils with antibacterial and antiviral actions, such as eucalyptus, tea tree, garlic, thyme, mixed with water and alcohol, can be sprayed into the airspace of stables and barns to reduce the risk of airborne infection.

An old-fashioned nosebag can be used for horses of all ages to help open up the airways, encourage expectoration and fight infection. Place a cotton gamgee-type pad in the base of a nosebag or grazing muzzle, and add a few drops of your chosen essential oil to the pad. The volatile oil molecules act on the sense of smell and affect mucous secretions of the respiratory system.

Choose oils such as pine, thyme, eucalyptus, garlic, peppermint, tea tree or Olbas.

Nature has provided us with literally dozens of herbs for the respiratory system, to encourage expectoration, soothe inflammation in the airways, reduce production of mucus or make it more watery and therefore easier to expel. In addition there are a number of herbs that offer specific action against viral or bacterial agents, such as *Strep* (*Streptococcus*), *Staph* (*Staphylococcus*), etc.

Depending on the nature of the problem, choose herbs from the following categories to help with a variety of respiratory problems. Remember that dried herbs will take several weeks to get into the system, so if you anticipate problems with either seasonal allergies or when the horse is stabled, start giving the herbs three to four weeks before the danger period.

Expectorants – these herbs increase bronchial mucus secretions by first making the mucus more liquid and then promoting its expulsion from the body. They have a secondary action of constricting blood vessels, which leads to a reduction of blood supply to the inflamed lining of the nasal passages. They include: aniseed, coltsfoot, comfrey, elderflower, hyssop, mullein, liquorice, thyme and garlic.

Refrigerants – these are herbs with a cooling effect that will reduce temperature and inflammation: plantain, marshmallow leaf, lemon balm and liquorice.

Anticatarrhals – generally, the production of catarrh is the body's way of dealing with allergies or infection, of both the upper and lower respiratory system. This system should not usually be interfered with. However, there are times when it can be helpful to reduce the amount of mucus being produced by the mucosal cells.

Plantain and eyebright are very specific for this; their astringent action will reduce secretion by the mucous membranes, and can be helpful for conditions such as hay fever or blocked sinuses. Both these plants contain a constituent called aucubin, which is thought to be antibacterial. Eyebright is the herb of choice for any sinus problems. It can also be used in solution for bathing sore or irritated eyes.

Plantain – rich in mucilage and containing the glycoside aucubin, which is both anti-catarrhal and antibiotic.

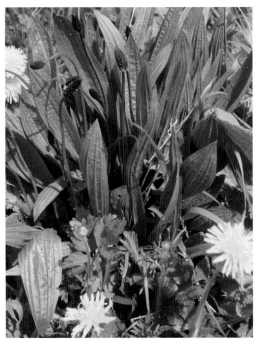

Mucilages – these are herbs that contain soothing, cooling mucilage, which will ease irritable tickly coughs, reduce inflammation and help relax spasms in the bronchials: marshmallow leaf, liquorice, plantain, comfrey and coltsfoot.

Febrifuge – these are herbs that will help to reduce a high temperature by increasing sweating and dilating the blood vessels in the skin, thereby allowing the heat to escape. A high temperature is always a cause for concern, so seek veterinary advice if you are worried. Febrifuges include: elderflowers, yarrow, boneset, peppermint, meadowsweet and willow.

Antihistamines – these are herbs that will lessen the severity of allergic reactions; they are non-sedating and can be used for seasonal allergic reactions: garlic, calendula, chamomile, marshmallow root, eyebright, echinacea, peppermint and nettle.

Bronchodilators – these are herbs that will dilate and open up the airways; they are good to use for severe allergic attacks, such as seasonal rhinitis: thyme, white horehound, peppermint and chamomile.

Antimicrobials – these are herbs that either destroy or inhibit the growth of disease-causing bacteria; many of them have been clinically proven to be effective against specific bacteria: thyme, garlic, calendula (specific against *E.coli*, *Staph* and *Strep*), echinacea, elecampane (specific against the TB bacillus), plantain, eyebright and sage.

Recent research carried out at the University of East London has confirmed that the allicin component of garlic is effective against even the notorious MRSA antibiotic-resistant 'superbug'. Fresh garlic cloves can be given to horses – 4–5 cloves daily; or use good quality garlic powder/granules to ensure a good allicin content.

Antivirals – these are herbs that have the ability to suppress the growth of viruses: elecampane, echinacea, elderflower, yarrow, liquorice and calendula. Calendula has been the subject of much research and has been found to have a strong antiviral activity against flu viruses.

It is interesting to note that several of the herbs such as liquorice, garlic, elderflower, plantain, yarrow, echinacea and calendula are mentioned in more than one category. This confirms the multifunctional nature of herbal medicine: that one plant can offer several different actions because of its various active constituents.

❧ Homeopathic Remedies

There are a number of remedies that are appropriate for coughs and seasonal allergies or that will encourage the loosening and expulsion of mucus.

The appropriate remedy is selected depending on the presenting symptoms. Consult a homeopathic vet or reference book to identify the most appropriate remedy for the horse.

Senega – for tough non-productive coughs.

Pulsatilla – for creamy mucus.

Phosphorus – for dry coughs, haemorrhage, epistaxis.

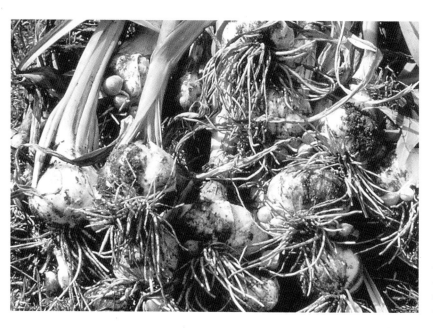

*Garlic – the 'superplant' whose extensive list of actions and benefits continue to be confirmed by modern medical research.
(Photo: McOnegal Botanical)*

✿ *Bach Flower Remedies*

Crab apple – for cleansing, if there is infection.

Rescue/Recovery Remedy – for distress caused by severe respiratory difficulties.

RHEUMATISM – SEE ARTHRITIS

SARCOIDS

These semi-malignant growths are thought to be viral in nature. They grow in a variety of sites and can break open and bleed if they are caught or rubbed. There are a number of conventional treatments available, but these can be expensive and painful. With the older horse in mind, I would certainly recommend trying herbal and/or homeopathic remedies before resorting to conventional treatments.

Sarcoids should be treated internally and externally, in the same way that you would tackle any other infection that has taken advantage of a lowered immune response. Strengthen the body and help it fight the invasion by feeding herbs with immune-strengthening, antiviral, antibacterial and 'anti-tumour' actions. Build up the horse's immunity so that the body is able to 'reject' the viral infection. Apply herbs topically, to reduce inflammation; use astringent herbs to stop bleeding and encourage healing of cells, and use plants with an antimitotic action to slow down cellular growth.

Be patient: sarcoids can take years to develop, so you must give the herbs time to work. I would give the herbs for at least three or four months. If possible, start during the winter months, when there is less risk of flies aggravating the sarcoid if it becomes sore or bloody. Sometimes the sarcoid can appear to get bigger as it is pushed out of the body – I take this as a good sign, and an indication that the body is rejecting the foreign object.

Herbs can also be used prophylactically. If, for example, the horse had a sarcoid removed by conventional treatment, herbs can be given to help prevent it returning. I spoke to one vet who told me that she had seen an X-ray of her horse's sarcoid, showing its rooting system, spreading over an area the size of her fist!

Antibacterial or antibiotic herbs: burdock, myrrh, echinacea, golden-seal, thyme, garlic, calendula, echinacea and cleaver.

Antivirals – these are herbs that have the ability to suppress the growth of viruses: burdock, echinacea, garlic, yarrow and liquorice.

Calendula – this plant has been the subject of much research and has been found to have a strong activity against the *Herpes simplex* virus.

Vitamin C has a broad spectrum action against viruses, so herbs or vegetables containing high levels of vitamin C should also be used, such as: rosehip, nettle, burdock and green leafy vegetables.

Immune system strengtheners – echinacea, cleaver and garlic.

Anti-tumour – the following herbs have all traditionally been used for their 'anti-cancer' properties: burdock, cleaver, calendula, garlic, echinacea, comfrey, dandelion, yellow dock, wormwood and fenugreek.

❀ *Topical Applications*

For topical application use a calendula cream base with the addition of distilled witch hazel and any of the following tinctures: thuja, echinacea, dandelion leaf, garlic, or greater celandine. Apply to the sarcoid at least twice a day.

❀ *Homeopathic Remedies*

There are several remedies that can help in the treatment of sarcoids. One is thuja, a traditional remedy for viral conditions such as warts and sarcoids. Consult your homeopathic vet or a good reference book for advice on the most appropriate remedy for your horse.

SCOURING – SEE DIGESTIVE DISORDERS

TEETH PROBLEMS

Oral hygiene, extraction, infection

Throughout this book, I have emphasised the need to check your horse's teeth regularly, because so many other problems can occur if the teeth are neglected. We have our horses' teeth checked by an equine dentist every

Use diluted sugar-beet water to encourage drinking. Use sugar-beet water and/or pulp to soften food and make it easier to chew. (Photo by Annie Dent)

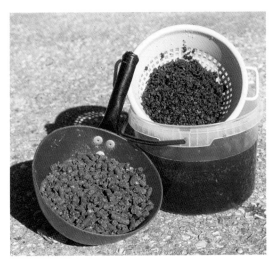

six months, but each horse is an individual and the condition of its teeth will vary.

As horses age, their teeth will deteriorate, the gums can recede and a condition known as periodontal pocketing may occur. This is when the gum that surrounds the tooth forms a pocket which traps food particles. The food becomes impacted between the gum and the tooth, providing an ideal environment for infection. The older horse may also struggle to deal with fibrous or unprocessed cereals, dropping food out of its mouth, dunking food or hay in the water bucket, or quidding. These are all signs of the horse having difficulty in chewing food and may indicate that horse is in pain. In these circumstances, take veterinary and equine dental advice as to what treatment is most appropriate for your horse's presenting dental condition.

Feeding steamed hay or haylage can help the older horse whose teeth are deteriorating. Feed can be softened or pre-soaked, using sugar-beet water or pulp. Chopped alfalfa is particularly nutritious and easier for the older horse to chew. In the past I have used soaked alfalfa cubes and pre-steamed linseed and fenugreek to help keep condition on an old horse, especially over the winter months.

When one of our horses was twenty-six he needed to have two teeth extracted from his lower jaw. Over the years his teeth had grown up out of the gum and the gum had receded. He ended up with the roots of the teeth poking out through the side of the gum. As you can imagine, this was not only extremely uncomfortable for him, but also led to inflammation of the gums, mouth ulcers and an infection caused by food becoming trapped.

I managed to clear up the mouth ulcers and infection using herbs with an antibacterial action. We brushed the area twice each day to help remove trapped food and gave him fresh garlic cloves twice a day. In addition I used herbs such as dandelion root, burdock, cleavers and echinacea, in conjunction with plenty of fresh fruit and vegetables, and a mouth-wash made from sage and tincture of myrrh.

Our vet administered a sedative, so the dentist would be able to extract the teeth without the risk of the horse throwing his head around. Immediately before the operation, and for several days after the extraction, I administered the homeopathic remedy arnica. This was to help with both the shock of the operation and reduce bruising to the gums and jaw. Immediately after the extraction I gave the homeopathic remedy Staphasagria. This remedy is used whenever there is surgical intervention. I also syringed distilled witch hazel mixed with a few drops of hypericum and calendula tincture, into the cavities to stop the bleeding, reduce pain and inflammation and promote healing. I continued to syringe this area of his mouth with the witch hazel mixture over the next five days and fed a variety of herbs with antiseptic and healing actions, such as thyme, sage, garlic and calendula.

SINUS INFECTIONS RELATED TO TOOTH PROBLEMS

Another condition that is worth mentioning here is the instance of sinus infections. I have heard of several horses presenting with repeated sinus infections. They would be given a course of antibiotics, which would clear up the condition, only for it to reappear a few weeks later. After the antibiotics failed to deal with the problem, the horses then had their sinuses

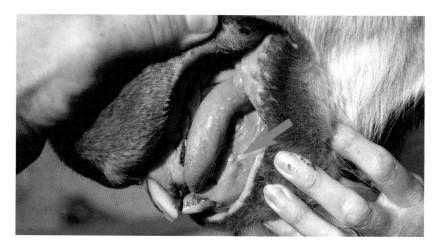

Site of tooth extraction. Note the well healed area and healthy gum.

flushed with antibacterial solutions, and some had the sinuses drilled and drained.

In several of these cases, the cause of the problem was eventually found to be an infected root of a tooth, that had affected the surrounding jaw bone. If, therefore, your horse is prone to repeated sinus infections, it is always worth having the teeth checked by a competent equine dentist, and if necessary, arranging for X-rays to be taken of the jaw.

ULCERATION – SEE DIGESTIVE DISORDERS

URINARY PROBLEMS

Infections, inflammation of the urinary tract, incontinence, kidney stones, bladder stones/gravel, reluctance to stale, painful urination

There are many herbs that can be used for urinary problems: diuretics, urinary antiseptics, antilithics, and demulcents.

Always check with your vet, and obtain a diagnosis to ascertain the cause of any urinary problem. This is vital in order to ensure the symptoms are not indicative of a more serious underlying condition. Oedema, infection, difficulty in urinating, blood in the urine, or painful urination can all be symptoms of more serious problems, such as heart or kidney disease, cancer or stones.

Important note: Some of the stronger urinary antiseptics should not be used if the horse has kidney disease, kidney failure or is pregnant. Long-term treatment with urinary antiseptics is not usually recommended. The cause of the infection should be identified and then treated.

URINARY INFECTION

With any urinary infection, the most important thing is to try to ensure the horse drinks as much water as possible. This will help flush the kidneys and will also carry the beneficial components of any herbal medicine through to the urinary system. To encourage horses to drink, add weak sugar-beet water or apple juice to the horse's water, and make feeds nice and wet.

Urinary infection, inflammation or a chill on the kidneys can lead to symptoms such as a reluctance to drop the penis, difficulty in urinating or pain on urination.

Diuretics – conventional modern diuretics work by increasing the flow of urine from the kidneys and thereby the expulsion of fluid from the body. The problem with some of these diuretics is that they will also increase the expulsion of electrolytes such as potassium and sodium from the body.

Herbs such as dandelion, nettle, birch, elder, chamomile and lime flowers contain high levels of potassium and can be used to help replace the potassium lost during diuresis. Herbal diuretics can be used to reduce oedema, fluid retention, inflammation of the kidneys or bladder, and to ensure that the inflammatory waste products of arthritis and rheumatism are excreted from the body.

Urinary antiseptics – herbs with a urinary antiseptic action generally contain essential oils, whose germicidal action will destroy harmful bacteria as they are excreted from the body via the kidneys, bladder and ureters.

These herbs often have a diuretic action that will increase the amount of fluid excreted by the kidneys. This action will put additional pressure on the kidneys. It is important, therefore, that you make sure the horse is not suffering from kidney disease before you administer these herbs.

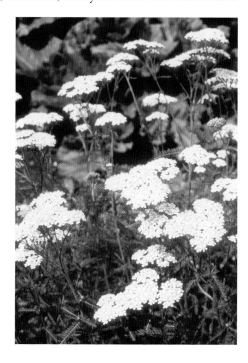

Urinary antiseptics include yarrow, buchu, golden-seal, saw palmetto and bearberry (the antiseptic action of bearberry depends on the urine being alkaline).

Meadowsweet can be used if there is infection in any area of the urinary system.

Yarrow – when there is blood in the urine then yarrow is specific because of its antihaemorrhagic action. Bear in mind that blood in the urine

Yarrow.
(Photo: McOnegal Botanical)

could indicate more serious conditions such as kidney/bladder stones.

Calendula – yeast infections can develop if the delicate balance of bacteria in the gut or urinary tract has been affected by antibiotic medication; calendula is the herb of choice for fungal, yeast, viral and bacterial infections of the urinary system.

Liquorice – it has been suggested that many of the bacteria responsible for urinary infections are successful because they have the ability to adhere to the smooth surface of the bladder and urinary tract. Liquorice is specific for bladder infections. Its demulcent action will help prevent bacteria from adhering to the bladder walls. In clinical trials the juice from bilberry, blueberry and cranberry fruits have also been shown to be able to interfere with this mechanism. This is why so many women find drinking real (not processed) cranberry juice so effective for cystitis.

Couch grass – the herb couch grass is an all-round urinary herb. It is little wonder that horses and dogs alike will eat this grass whenever they have the opportunity. In herbal medicine the roots of the plant are used. Couch grass has both a diuretic and demulcent action and is good for conditions such as urethritis, cystitis, gall and kidney stones.

Golden rod is a herb with a specific affinity for the kidneys. It is diuretic, anti-inflammatory, antiseptic to mucous membranes, and supports the fine micro-capillary system of the kidneys. I use golden rod for Cushing's disease in order to support the kidneys, which are under pressure due to polyuria.

Urinary Inflammation

Where there is infection there will inevitably be inflammation, which can lead to: reluctance to urinate, retained urine or a reluctance to drop the penis fully and stale properly. Herbs with a gentle demulcent action will reduce inflammation in the urinary tract, by soothing and protecting the inflamed mucous membrane. Use herbs such as couch grass, liquorice, marshmallow leaf and corn silk in conjunction with appropriate urinary antiseptics.

Incontinence

The causes of incontinence are many and can include nerve damage, muscle weakness, loss of tone in the bladder sphincter, injury and degeneration of the spinal cord.

Urinary astringents, such as plantain and calendula, can be used to help tighten up a sphincter muscle that may have lost tone; while herbs such as corn silk are recommended for an uncontrollable bladder.

❧ Bach Flower Remedies

Aspen – for a weak bladder.

Crab apple – for inner cleansing and infection.

Cherry plum – for loss of control of urination.

Urinary Stones or Gravel

These do not appear to be a common condition, but some horses seem to be prone to developing stones or gravel in the kidneys or bladder. Over time they can become large and painful, and if in the kidneys can lead to renal colic. Horses can present with pain on urination, reluctance to urinate, incomplete urination, blood in the urine, hollowing of the back during urination, erection or symptoms of a chill on the kidneys. These symptoms could also indicate cystitis or urethritis, so make sure you get this checked out before assuming the horse has stones!

Attention to the diet in susceptible horses is important as cereal consumption, mineral deficiency, digestive disorders or long-term treatment for ulceration have all been linked to an increase in the risk of stone formation.

Surgery is sometimes necessary, but the use of herbal antilithics and demulcents can help with the dissolution and elimination of stones or gravel, if not too large. These same herbs can also be used prophylactically to help prevent the formation of stones.

Golden rod is a herb with a special affinity for the kidneys. It is reputed to be able to help decrease kidney and bladder stones.

Antilithics – these are herbs that have the ability to help break up or dissolve kidney or bladder stones. They are a long-term treatment and should be used in conjunction with demulcent herbs.

Gravel root – I have used this herb prophylactically in a mix for a vet whose client's horse had a propensity to develop stones. Gravel root contains volatile oils and resins, and is also a diuretic.

Wild hydrangea – diuretic and contains volatile oils.

Urinary demulcents – These herbs will soothe and protect the irritated and inflamed mucous membrane of the urinary tract. They are particularly indicated for urinary-tract infections and stones. Their key constituent is mucilage.

Marshmallow leaf – this herb is ideal for inflammatory urinary conditions and cystitis.

Couch grass – this herb contains the constituent mannitol, which has an antibiotic action.

Plantain – rich in mucilage, soothing and healing; contains the glycoside aucubin, which is antibiotic.

Corn silk – diuretic and specific for urethritis, prostatitis and cystitis.

SHEATH CLEANING

This is a good opportunity to mention the cleaning of a horse's sheath. As horses age there may be a risk of growths developing on the outside of the penis. These can become irritated and sore as the horse draws the penis in and out to urinate.

Horses can also develop melanomas high up inside the sheath, which may break open periodically. I have seen some horses plagued with flies in the summer when the sarcoids on their penis or teats have become rubbed and sore. See the appropriate sections for suggestions on which herbs to give internally.

Externally you can use a soothing antiseptic wash to help cleanse these areas, reduce the greasiness, and offer some antiseptic action to help prevent the spread of infection.

To help reduce itching, inflammation or discomfort, make an infusion using herbs such as: marshmallow root, chamomile, lady's mantle, calendula or St John's wort.

If the area is infected then make an infusion using echinacea, calendula or golden-seal.

To help break down excessive grease (smegma) use astringents such as witch hazel or diluted cider vinegar.

These teas can be used to bathe the area, or sprayed onto the penis via a spray bottle if this is easier. See the section on herbal preparations for instructions.

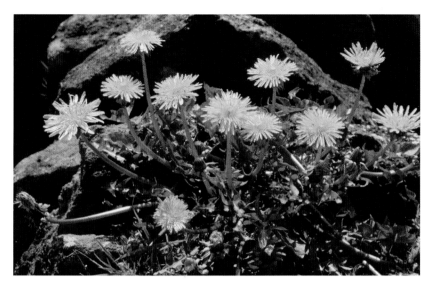

Dandelion, also known as 'pee-the-bed' – nature's finest diuretic.

Note: It is important to strike a happy medium regarding sheath cleaning. Over-cleaning of the sheath, particularly with strong antiseptics such as iodine, can upset the natural balance of flora allowing opportunist organisms such as yeasts to flourish.

✿ *Homeopathic Remedies*

There are specific remedies for growths, abscesses or tumours that grow where the mucous membrane meets the outside skin such as around the anus or on the penis. Consult a homeopathic vet for advice on the best remedy.

WEIGHT LOSS – SEE DIGESTIVE DISORDERS, AND

APPETITE, LACK OF

❀

CHAPTER THREE

Wounds and First Aid

THIS SECTION CONTAINS suggestions for the management and care of minor wounds, bruises and scrapes. Seek veterinary attention for any serious injuries and deep wounds.

First-aid attention within any stable management is important; with the older horse, however, it is even more vital that any wound or injury receives prompt attention.

As horses age, wound healing can become slower, skin is thinner and less resistant, horses may bruise more easily and the immune response may be lowered. If a condition such as Cushing's disease exists, then the horse may be even more likely to suffer from repeated infections.

I have already discussed the importance of supporting the veteran horse's immunity with herbs that will help strengthen the immune response to injury and infection.

MINOR WOUNDS

For small cuts and abrasions a soothing antiseptic spray can be made using aloe vera and/or witch hazel as a base. Witch hazel is an excellent astringent and ideal for use on bruises, swellings or minor scrapes. Aloe vera is a cleanser and will promote healing.

To this base add herbs with antiseptic and cleansing actions to reduce inflammation and encourage healing of the wound, such as: echinacea, hypericum, comfrey, garlic, calendula, golden-seal, gotu kola or plantain. This mix can be placed in a hand-held spray and misted onto the wound, regardless of its location. The mix is also water-soluble, and can be easily irrigated out of the wound if veterinary attention is needed.

If a wound has become infected, or if there is pus present, then echinacea, myrrh or golden-seal with their antiseptic, antifungal and anti-inflammatory actions should be considered.

Herbs should be used both topically and internally, to support the body and encourage granulation of tissue and cell proliferation.

Internally use plants such as seaweed, calendula, cleaver, garlic, burdock, echinacea.

Comfrey leaf, and gotu kola both have the ability to accelerate cell division and speed up the healing of wounds. They are particularly effective for healing of mucous membrane, and can be used both internally and externally.

Feed fresh vegetables and fruits rich in vitamin C, to increase the horse's resistance to infection. Vitamin E can help to dissolve blood clots, and can encourage healing without scarring. Herbs such as oats, kelp, dandelion leaves, fenugreek, and leafy green vegetables are rich in vitamin E, as well as oils such as soya, wheatgerm and corn.

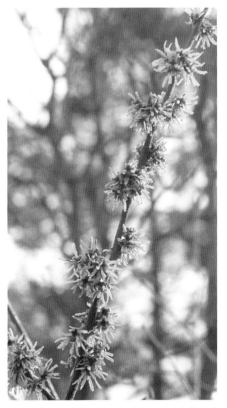

Above: Witch hazel.
(Photo: McOnegal Botanical)

Below: Comfrey.

Bruising

Horses will be horses, and it is a fairly safe bet that if a horse sustains an injury there will also be bruising to the area.

Comfrey is the supreme herb for bruising. I always keep a comfrey compress in the first-aid kit. Use comfrey for bruising, bowed and sprained tendons, or as a poultice to help draw out pus.

Calendula and chamomile are good to use if the skin has been abraded or chaffed. The flowers are antiseptic, anti-inflammatory and will reduce pain in superficial wounds.

Echinacea stimulates circulation, which will encourage healing.

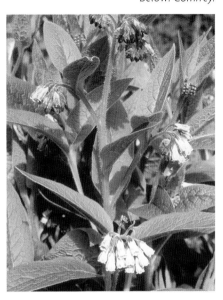

Arnica tincture is excellent for bruising, but do not use it on open wounds.

Note: Spontaneous bruising may be an indication of a more serious condition, so contact your vet if this occurs.

POULTICES

See the section on herb preparations and applications for details on how to prepare a poultice or compress.

Nature has provided us with a number of herbs that make excellent poultices. These can be used to help draw abscesses and infection, encourage the removal of foreign objects from the body (such as thorns), ulceration or wounds.

Slippery elm powder and marshmallow root powder make fantastic poultice bases. They are herbs that are traditionally used when a 'drawing' action is required. They both contain mucilage which, with its soothing and healing properties, will encourage the removal of pus from boils and abscesses. Other herbs can be added to the slippery elm or marshmallow base, depending on what the problem is. Nowadays, adhesive dressings are available that will stick to the horse's coat, making it much easier to apply a poultice or compress to areas that are difficult to bandage.

For ulceration, use comfrey root, seaweed or honey.

For wounds that refuse to heal, use comfrey, echinacea, gotu kola and aloe vera.

For infection use burdock, golden-seal, echinacea and myrrh.

For drawing abscesses, and foreign objects such as thorns, use slippery elm, marshmallow root, comfrey, plantain, mullein or cleaver.

Note: I used a burdock and slippery elm poultice on a leg that had become infected and refused to heal. Burdock is known as the 'power digger' of the herb world for its ability to 'draw' poisons and waste products out of the cells. I poulticed the leg four times, by which time the infection had cleared and the skin was looking pink and healthy again. I then used gotu kola compresses to encourage tissue renewal.

COMPRESSES

These are used externally to help soften tissue, reduce inflammation or alleviate pain. Use herbs or essential oils (suitably diluted), depending on what you are dealing with.

For bleeding or bruising, use witch hazel, yarrow, comfrey root, or arnica tincture (but do not use arnica on open wounds).

For inflammation use calendula, chamomile tincture or essential oil, hypericum tincture or essential oil (particularly for areas where there are lots of nerve endings).

For pain, use rosemary essential oil, chamomile tincture or essential oil, or hypericum tincture or essential oil.

For infection, use golden-seal, echinacea, myrrh; a few drops of Bach Flower crab apple remedy can also be added.

CREAMS AND OINTMENTS

Natural plant-based creams, ointments and balms are now much more readily available. These creams containing plant extracts and/or essential oils can be applied to minor cuts and abrasions. Comfrey, calendula or chickweed are often used in a base cream, to which tinctures or oils such as hypericum, garlic, chamomile, etc. are added to provide an anti-inflammatory, soothing and healing action.

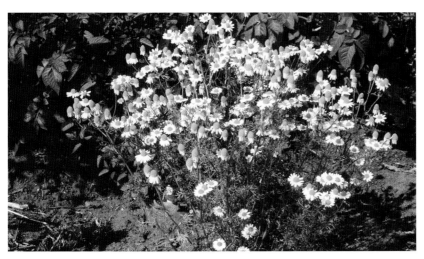

Chamomile. (Photo: McOnegal Botanical)

Honey has been used for centuries as a natural product to encourage healing of ulcers and wounds that refuse to mend. It is both cooling and analgesic. Smear a dressing or gauze pad with honey and use on cuts, scratches, bites, stings or boils. Honey will inhibit the growth of bacteria, speed up granulation and has been found to arrest necrotic tissue. If you are going to use honey make sure that it is good quality (preferably organic); some of the cheaper, more processed honeys are often sourced from several different countries and do not contain the same properties.

✿ *Homeopathic Remedies*

Arnica – for shock and bruising.

Hypericum – for painful wounds and nerve endings.

Hepar sulph – for suppurating infected wounds; it will reduce the risk of infection following injury. This remedy is also good for abscesses that have not yet come to a head.

Silica – for chronic infections, abscesses and to help resolve scar tissue. Use for infected discharging wounds where pus is draining well, and to assist in the rejection of foreign material from the body.

Calendula – to promote healing of any wound; particularly good for painful wounds, lacerations and cuts.

Euphrasia – this remedy can be used for conjunctivitis and other eye infections or wounds. Use a few doses of arnica first, for any injuries associated with the eye and surrounding area.

✿ *Bach Flower Remedies*

Rescue/Recovery Remedy – should be kept in the first-aid kit and used whenever accidents occur. Use on both the horse and the rider/handler.

Crab apple – for infection, abscesses and wounds.

Rescue/Recovery Cream – can be used for wounds, particularly where there has been trauma.

❀

CHAPTER FOUR

The Older Horse's Diet, and Worming

A horse's diet is a specialist subject and one that I am not qualified to advise on. That said, obviously an older horse will need a different diet from that of a younger horse working or competing regularly. I would suggest that you contact a reputable feed company, or an independent nutritionist to obtain advice on the best feed for your horse. This will be based on how much work the horse is doing, what the pasture is like, how long the horse is out at grass, and what type of hay/haylage is being fed.

Just on a general note, as with any horse, the diet should include as much access to grazing as possible, good quality forage, and plenty of fresh fruit and vegetables. (I feed the following fruits and vegetables to our horses: carrots, apples, pears, peas, cabbage, cauliflower stalks, celery, broccoli, parsnips, and swede.) It is particularly important for the older horse to keep moving and get its head down; this helps stretch and relax muscles, promotes good circulation and helps keep the airways clear of mucus. Try to place all feed (coarse mix, haylage, hay, etc.) on the ground or floor of the stable, as this encourages the horse to drop its head.

A plentiful supply of clean water is, of course, vital and food should be fed little and often. The diet should include plenty of long fibre, and an easily digestible energy source.* Many feed manufacturers are now producing mixes formulated specifically for veteran horses. Most feeds these days contain a balanced vitamin and mineral supply, but check with a

---

* If using a feed containing oil, check the source of the oil. Many high-fat equine feeds use animal fats, which are high in saturated fats, as an energy source.

nutritionist on any specific requirements for the older horse. A shortage, or excess, of some minerals and vitamins can lead to ill health and the appearance of clinical symptoms. It is important to remember that however good the horse's diet is, it will only be of benefit if the digestive system is functioning correctly and effectively.

Prebiotics and Probiotics – What Are They?

I have already mentioned the use of prebiotics and probiotics in several other sections, but there are still many people who are not familiar with their actions or applications. The equine gut contains a vast quantity of bacteria – beneficial and not so beneficial – that generally live in peaceful co-existence. These bacteria help to maintain the correct pH levels in the system, assist in the break down of fibre, and help in the synthesis of vitamins such as biotin. Sometimes this delicate balance can be upset, allowing the not-so-beneficial bacteria to flourish at the expense of the beneficial ones. This upset in the gut flora can lead to digestive disorders, poor absorption of nutrients, inflammation and scouring. It is at times like these that a prebiotic and a probiotic can help.

Prebiotics

In essence, probiotics restore the levels of beneficial bacteria in the gut, whereas prebiotics feed existing beneficial bacteria.

A prebiotic is a non-digestible food that selectively stimulates the growth of beneficial bacteria that already exist in the gut. In human trials, plants containing fructo-oligosaccharides (FOSs) have proved to be effective prebiotics. This is because FOSs are not destroyed or absorbed as they pass through the first part of the digestive system, so they are still viable when they reach the gut. Plants containing these FOSs include: garlic, onions, oats, soya beans and Jerusalem artichokes.

Probiotics

A probiotic is a collection of beneficial bacteria. When you use a probiotic, you are providing a dose of live bacteria, to help replenish the levels of the beneficial bacteria in the gut. There are now several commercially available probiotics that have been specifically formulated for equine use. Ensure that the probiotic you use contains bacteria indigenous to the equine digestive system, such as: *Enterococcus faecium, Lactobacillus casei* or *Lactobacillus acidophilus.* These bacteria will help to redress the imbalance and get things on an even keel again.

One of the simplest (although not as effective as a specific probiotic) products that can be used as a probiotic, is organic 'live' yoghurt. This is readily available in most supermarkets and can either be added to feed or syringed into the mouth. I like to give it in conjunction with a good dollop of honey.

I give our horses a probiotic mixed with powdered herbs such as marshmallow root, garlic and slippery elm. The probiotic replenishes the good bacteria, while the herbs reduce inflammation and ease cramping of the smooth muscle in the gut wall. Garlic is a natural pro- and prebiotic, and has been shown to be effective against many of the coliforms and anaerobes found in faeces.

WHEN TO USE A PRE- OR PROBIOTIC

- After the use of antibiotics – there is no point giving the probiotic while the horse is on antibiotics as the drug will negate the beneficial effects.

- In conjunction with any other medication.

- Prior to, during and after travelling.

- Whenever there is a change of diet.

- In conjunction with, and after using conventional wormers.

- At any time of stress.

- To both the mare and foal during foal heat.

- If the horse has diarrhoea or even overly soft droppings.

HANDY TIP

Use a probiotic and the herb milk thistle when you are administering a conventional wormer. The probiotic will help restore the gut bacteria destroyed by the wormer and the milk thistle will help support and protect the liver from the chemicals in the system.

Worming and Parasitism

As horses age, their immunity and therefore their resistance to parasites may be lowered. This can lead to an unthrifty look and failure to thrive. Needless to say, good horse management includes not only an appropriate worming programme, but also attention to pasture maintenance and care. In the wild, horses graze and then move on, leaving their dung- and urine-soiled areas behind them. In captivity this is not possible, but even so, horses will develop dedicated areas where they stale and dung in order to keep parasites away from their grazing areas. Nature's pharmacy has provided us with a large number of natural anthelmintics, vermicides and vermifuges that will help destroy and expel worms. In the wild there is extensive evidence of animals seeking out anthelmintic plants and self-dosing, particularly at critical times such as when the parasites are migrating. These observations confirm the herbal tradition of administering anthelmintic plants when the moon is waxing (just before the full moon) because this is the time when parasites tend to migrate.

Many of the herbs used for their antiparasitic action are powerful purgatives, so care should always be taken when using herbal wormers. By their very nature, herbal anthelmintics are 'toxic' in that they create an environment that is harmful to parasites. Therefore a delicate balance

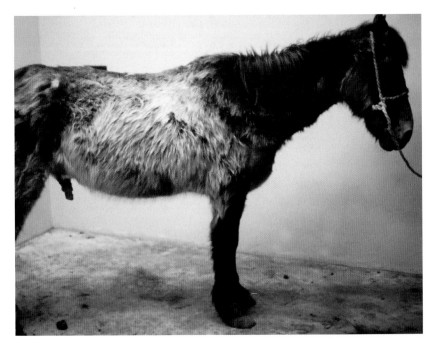

This poor pony was diagnosed with chronic parasitism, but was later discovered to be suffering from poor teeth. (Photo courtesy of R. Fisher BVetSc, MRCVS)

HANDY TIPS

Use grated carrots and seeds such as milk thistle, pumpkin, melon, pomegranate and sunflower to help scour the gut wall and create an inhospitable environment for worms.

In her book *Wild Health*, Cindy Engel writes of a group of chimpanzees that deliberately fold and swallow leaves with rough and barbed surfaces. When the excreted leaves were examined in the faeces, they were found to have worms attached to the tiny barbs. This is an example of how animals deliberately ingest plants to help with the mechanical expulsion of parasites. Horses will go to no end of trouble and will risk having their tender muzzles pricked by vicious thorns in order to collect the seeds contained in thistle heads. Is this another example of self medication?

If your horse is looking poor or 'wormy' don't automatically assume that parasites are the cause. The photograph on the facing page shows a very poor and sickly looking pony that had originally been diagnosed with chronic parasitism. On closer examination, however, it was discovered that the pony's problems were due entirely to the lamentable condition of its teeth!

I make no apology for returning to the subject of teeth – they are at the very beginning of the digestive system, and if neglected can have an enormous impact on a horse's health.

must be struck between using enough herbs to kill or eliminate the parasites, but not so much that the horse will be harmed. All herbalists recommend that doses of anthelmintic plants should be given in conjunction with herbs that soothe the digestive system (marshmallow root, slippery elm, liquorice), reduce any griping or smooth muscle spasm (valerian, mint, cramp bark, chamomile), and then help encourage the elimination of the parasites with their laxative action (dandelion root, aloe vera, plantain, yellow dock).

Note: Several anthelmintic herbs contain thujone which is contraindicated in pregnancy.

Garlic – is the supreme wormer; its volatile oil contains allicin which has been clinically proven to be effective against common intestinal parasites such as nematodes (roundworm).

Southernwood – this plant is effective again nematodes; it contains thujone.

Wormwood – this also contains thujone and is effective against nematodes and ascarids.

Mugwort – contains thujone; it can be used for all worm types but is weaker than wormwood and southernwood.

Elecampane – effective against threadworm.

Tansy – contains thujone; is effective against threadworm and roundworm.

Thyme – contains the volatile oil thymol, which is antiseptic, antibacterial and anthelmintic.

❖

CHAPTER FIVE

The Veteran Competitor

THIS BOOK would not be complete without a mention of the veteran competitor. My Lusitano gelding's insurance has just come up for renewal, and the insurance company have designated him as a veteran at the age of fifteen! I am fully anticipating he could live to at least thirty, which means that he is only half way through his life. It's just as well that life insurance companies don't apply the same criteria to humans, or we wouldn't be able to get any medical insurance or life cover after the age of thirty-six!

I am thinking of having him broken to harness, and would certainly consider competing him in years to come. One only has to see the success of the veteran golf and tennis tournaments to see how important it is to keep up the fitness, and provide both people and animals with a reason to get up every morning!

There are numerous examples of horses that continue to compete successfully, well into their twenties. Certainly in the sport of endurance it is not unusual to hear of a twenty-plus-year-old horse successfully completing an 80 or 100 mile ride, and easily satisfying the strict veterinary criteria.

The older horse has much to offer. With the benefit of years of experience, they are excellent companions and teachers for younger horses learning their trade. If care is taken in the early years there is no reason why horses in all disciplines shouldn't compete well into their late teens or twenties. These horses may not be as fast as they once were, and their recovery rates may not be as swift, but to the novice rider a schoolmaster is worth his or her weight in gold!

Obviously veteran competitors will require that bit more help if they are to cope with the rigours of the competitive world. More preparation may be needed, and additional effort given to ensure they are in the best possible condition.

The older horse cannot be expected to accomplish the physical extremes it achieved in its youth. More time will need to be allocated, in order to warm up older muscles prior to competition. Muscles and joints will benefit from regular passive stretching exercises, which can be made more fun with the use of carrots or treats as a reward. There are a number of excellent books now available with details of passive exercise regimes.

An older horse will find it harder to replace the electrolytes lost during effort. The kidneys, which are responsible for retaining electrolytes, are not as efficient, and potassium and sodium may be lost in the urine. Electrolytes should also be considered for use during training, and must always be used prior to, during and after competition. Weak sugar-beet water can be helpful in encouraging a horse to drink, during and after the competition to reduce the risk of dehydration.

These days, temporary stables are commonplace at competition venues, but they do tend to be relatively small. I would suggest that you should resist the temptation to leave the horse in his stable to 'relax', and instead make sure he has every opportunity to be walked out in hand. This will help prevent stiffening of joints and encourage the removal of waste products from the muscles. Needless to say, you will not want to walk the horse all night, so for the stabled period you could consider using a magnetic blanket or leg wraps. These items are invaluable for keeping old muscles and joints warm and supple. In addition, you could give your horse a good massage with a lotion containing essential oils (such as rosemary or lavender), and arnica tincture to stimulate circulation, warm the muscles and help clear lactic acid. Be aware that some essential oils contain substances that may be prohibited in competition.

For legs that have worked hard, apply cooling gels, clay or distilled witch hazel with arnica, willow and meadowsweet tincture. Support for tired legs is vital, and this can be achieved simply by bandaging with thick stable bandages to optimise blood circulation. Arnica tincture and witch hazel can be added to the wash-down water to reduce bruising and inflammation of the large muscle masses.

If the horse has sustained an injury during competition, a cleansing and antiseptic spray can be made using aloe vera gel mixed with witch hazel, hypericum, echinacea and calendula tinctures. Remember that arnica tincture should not be used on open wounds, and never used internally. Only homeopathic arnica should be given internally.

Recovery after competition will be slower for the older horse, and this is where herbs with an adaptogenic action are worth considering. Adaptogens are plants that assist the body's own regenerative powers, helping it to cope and recover from stress and support the natural immune response to additional effort.

Some of the adaptogens (such as the ginsengs) may be too stimulatory. I like to use the adaptogenic herb withania. I find it very appropriate for the elderly, in that it is stimulating, without putting additional strain on the body. I use withania for recovery from injury, convalescence after illness and for the older competitor.

Healthy and efficient lungs are vital for any competitor, and these organs must be kept in prime condition if you wish to continue competing your veteran horse. Lowered immunity in the older horse can increase the risk of infection or allergic reactions, and will result in a compromised respiratory system.

Ensure that the hay/haylage you feed is of the very best quality and dust free. Spray the stable, horsebox, trailer and temporary stabling at venues with an alcohol-based spray containing antiviral and antibacterial essential oils such as rosemary, thyme, tea tree and eucalyptus, to reduce the spread of airborne bacterial or viral infection.

If you are staying away from home, find out what type of bedding will be available at the venue, and take your own if the one provided is not suitable. Just one night in a stable with the wrong bedding can result in coughing and respiratory distress.

Any form of stress, such as travelling, competition or change of environment, will have an impact on the gut bacteria. Use a good probiotic before, during and after competition. Herbs that will help with digestion and reduce inflammation in the gut can be given in conjunction with the probiotics (see the section on digestive disorders and Chapter 4).

❀ *Homeopathic Remedies*

Arnica – bruising, shock.

Rhus tox – inflammation.

Ruta grav – sprains and strains.

Nux vomica – digestive upsets.

❀ *Bach Flower Remedies*

Walnut – this remedy should be used routinely for animals and people who have to deal with any sort of life changes, e.g. competition, travelling, change of home or stable yard, etc.

Olive – for revitalisation; this remedy should be used during and after competition to help restore mental and physical energy. Give to both horse and rider.

Rescue/Recovery Remedy – the all-purpose comforter, to help horse and rider cope with the stresses and strains of competition.

❖

CHAPTER SIX

The Final Chapter

I T IS A FACT OF LIFE that none of us lives forever. As William Shake-speare said in 1609: 'By medicine life may be prolonged, yet death will seize the doctor too.'

Taking the decision to let an old horse go has got to be one of the hardest choices that some of us will ever be asked to make. Nothing I can say will make it any easier, but I like to think that this is one thing we can do for the animals in our care, to ensure that they do not suffer unnecessarily and that they die with dignity. Viewed in this way, the decision may be somewhat easier to bear.

Each of us will deal with this difficult time in our own way. How you cope with it is up to you, and I would not presume to advise. I would recommend, though, that it is worthwhile thinking about what you want to do in advance and then make some preliminary arrangements. Sometimes, despite the best laid plans, events can overtake you, and you may find that once your horse is dead you are not able to deal with it in the way you would have liked.

I heard recently of someone whose horse was being looked after in another country where the owner used to live. The horse died suddenly and the body was dealt with before the owner could contact anyone to ask for a piece of the horse's mane to be kept for her. Obviously the owner was upset by the death of her horse, but even more upset that she had been unable to obtain this final keepsake.

Investigate the options for dealing with your horse before the time comes to make that final decision.

BURIAL

Some people are in the fortunate position of having their own land on which (local bylaws and services permitting) they can have their horse buried. In cases like this it is always worth contacting a local builder or farmer beforehand to make sure that they will be able to come over with a digger when the time comes. Obviously you will need to choose a burial site that can be easily accessed by the digger.

CREMATION

In the UK you can have your horse cremated and then scatter the ashes in an appropriate spot. There are a number of companies who can make the arrangements for you, and many of them advertise in the equestrian press. It is worth contacting them in advance, just to talk through what will need to be done when the time comes.

Some people like to keep a piece of their horse's mane or tail and then have it inset into a piece of jewellery. Others like to plant a tree in remembrance of their horse, pet or loved one.

The International League for the Protection of Horses (ILPH) offers a Tree of Remembrance Scheme. This was started in 2000 as a Millennium project, but continued due to the success of the scheme. The trees are planted at the charity's welfare centre in Norfolk, where the trees provide a natural windbreak and shelter from the weather for rescued horses. There is a minimum contribution (currently £30), which buys you a native species tree, with a small plaque on which can be noted the name of the horse, a short message and the name of the person sponsoring the tree.

I think this is a lovely idea. It helps protect the rescued horses, makes a contribution to a worthwhile charity and puts something back into the environment. Of course, there is nothing to stop you planting your own tree in your horse's paddock by way of a memorial.

Sometimes the decision will be taken out of your hands, and the horse will die of natural causes. Even so, it is always worth discussing with your vet in advance exactly how you want to deal with your horse when the time comes.

Those that are left behind

It is said that, unlike donkeys, horses do not make life-long friends. I would dispute this statement. I have certainly seen horses who, having lost long-term companions, displayed all the symptoms of depression and grief that we associate with the loss of a friend. Unfortunately I am not able to offer a magic potion for this situation. Time is a great healer and other companions can help to lessen the loss. What I can do is to recount the story of how we dealt with the situation when the time came for us to put my husband's old horse Ditton to sleep.

As I mentioned in an earlier section, Ditton had very bad melanomas. At the age of twenty-nine he started to lose co-ordination and proprio-ception of his back legs. Our vet had confirmed Ditton had melanomas internally, and that it was likely these had grown to such an extent that they were pressing on the spinal cord, causing him to lose proprioception. We were advised that there was nothing more that could be done and it was likely the horse's co-ordination would continue to deteriorate, leading to falls. Ditton was a big horse of 17.2hh; he had led a full and active life, and we were not prepared to see him lose his dignity or suffer from repeated falls due to this loss of awareness.

We had already decided that when the time came we would ask the vet to administer a lethal injection, and that we would have Ditton buried in our woods. It was a lovely day, and we walked Ditton slowly over to the woods with another horse who had been his companion for the previous ten years. With his friend grazing beside him the vet gave the injection, and in a very short time Ditton lay down and passed away peacefully.

Throughout this time his friend continued to graze just a few metres away from him. Needless to say, both my husband and I were pretty upset, and we stayed with Ditton for some time after he had died. Before taking our other horse back to the stables we led him over to Ditton's body, which he first sniffed and then felt gently all over with his muzzle. He then gave just one whinny, as if to say goodbye to his old friend for the last time.

Before going over to the woods, we had given both of the horses and ourselves the Bach Flower Remedy walnut. This is the remedy to use for helping both animals and people adapt to major changes in their lives. It is a remedy that should be used before and after anaesthesia and before euthanasia.

When we got back to the stables, and for several days afterwards, we continue to use the Bach Remedies of walnut and star of Bethlehem to help deal with the sadness and changes in our life. I am happy to say that, although our other horse was slightly at a loss for a few days, he seemed to cope well with the passing of his friend, and shortly afterwards teamed up with another of our horses for company.

✿ *Bach Flower Remedies*

Mustard – for depression; it restores serenity and dispels gloominess.

Walnut – for helping adapt to major life changes.

Star of Bethlehem – for shock, trauma and grief.

Rescue/Recovery Remedy – all-purpose comforter to reduce stress in any situation.

MATERIA MEDICA

The following list identifies all the plants I have mentioned in the book. Local names for plants can vary depending on which country or even which region you are in. For example, the plant *Galium aparine* is known as couch grass, catch grass, cleavers, clivers, sticky willy or sweethearts, depending on where in the UK you live.

Many people think that herbalists are just trying to impress when they refer to plants by their Latin names, but the reason they do this is in order to avoid any confusion with identification. If you intend collecting your own plant material and are unsure of a plant's identity, always consult a good reference book containing clear illustrations to make sure you get the right plant. The innocuous cow parsley, so loved by all our horses, can look very similar to the deadly hemlock.

Aloe vera – *Aloe vera*
Aniseed – *Pimpinella anisum*
Arnica – *Arnica montana*
Artichoke – *Cynara scolymus*
Bearberry – *Arctostaphylos uva ursi.*
Bilberry fruit – *Vaccinium myrtillis*
Boneset – *Eupatorium perfoliatum*
Buchu – *Barosma betulina*
Burdock – *Arctium lappa*
Buckwheat – *Fagopyrum esculentum*
Calendula – *Calendula officinalis*
Cayenne – *Capsicum minimum*
Celandine, Greater – *Chelidonium majus*
Celery seed – *Apium graveolens*
Chamomile – *Camomilla recutita, or Matricaria recutita*
Chaste tree – *Vitex agnus castus*
Chickweed – *Stellaria media*
Clary sage – *Salvia sclarea*
Cleavers – *Galium aparine*
Comfrey – *Symphytum officinale*
Corn silk – *Zea mays*

Couch grass – *Elymus repens*
Cramp bark – *Viburnum opulus*
Coltsfoot – *Tussilago farfara*
Dandelion leaf – *Taraxacum officinalis (folia)*
Dandelion root – *Taraxacum officinalis (radix)*
Devil's claw – *Harpagophytum procumbens*
Echinacea – *Echinacea species*
Elderflower – *Sambucus nigra*
Elecampane – *Inula helenium*
Eucalyptus – *Eucalyptus globulus*
Eyebright – *Euphrasia officinalis*
Fenugreek – *Trigonella foenum-graecum*
Fennel – *Foeniculum vulgare*
Garlic – *Allium sativum*
Ginger – *Zingiber officinale*
Ginkgo – *Ginkgo biloba*
Goat's rue – *Galega officinalis*
Golden rod – *Solidago virgaurea*
Golden-seal – *Hydrastis canadensis*
Gotu kola – *Centella asiatica*
Gravel root – *Eupatorium purpureum*
Hawthorn – *Crataegus oxyacantha*
Horehound – *Marrubium vulgare*
Hyssop – *Hyssopus officinalis*
Lady's mantle – *Alchemilla vulgaris*
Lavender – *Lavendula officinalis*
Lemon balm – *Melissa officinalis*
Liquorice – *Glycyrrhiza glabra*
Lovage – *Levisticum officinale*
Marigold – *Calendula officinalis*
Marshmallow root – *Althea officinalis (radix)*
Marshmallow leaf – *Althea officinalis (folia)*
Meadowsweet – *Filipendula ulmaria*
Milk thistle – *Silybum marianum*
Mint – *Mentha piperita*

Monk's pepper – *Vitex agnus castus*
Mullein – *Verbascum thapsus*
Myrrh – *Comiphora molmol*
Nettle – *Urtica dioica*
Oats – *Avena sativa*
Peppermint – *Mentha piperita*
Plantain – *Plantago lanceolata*
Prickly ash – *Zanthoxylum americanum*
Rosehip – *Rosa canina*
Rosemary – *Rosmarinus officinalis*
St John's wort – *Hypericum perforatum*
Saw palmetto – *Serenoa serrulata*
Seaweed – *Fucus vesiculosis*
Tea tree – *Melaleuca alternifolia*
Thuja – *Thuja occidentalis*
Thyme – *Thymus vulgaris*
Turmeric – *Curcuma longa*
Valerian – *Valeriana officinalis*
Wild hydrangea – *Hydrangea arborescens*
Willow – *Salix species*
Witch hazel – *Hamamelis virginiana*
Withania – *Withania somnifera*
Yarrow – *Achillea millefolium*
Yellow dock – *Rumex crispus*

GLOSSARY

Allergic rhinitis – an allergic condition with hypersensitivity of eyes, nose, throat and sometimes the skin due to grass and flower pollens.

Allopathic – the treatment of disease by conventional means (i.e. drugs).

Alterative – this is an old-fashioned term, which has more recently been superseded by the term 'blood purifier'. Alteratives will speed up tissue renewal.

Analgesic – pain relieving.

Anthelmintic – an agent that will cause the death, elimination or expulsion of worms and parasites.

Antibacterial – helps the body resist or destroy pathogenic micro-organisms.

Antibiotic/anti-infective – having the action of helping the body withstand infection or infestation. Note: some essential oils and cider vinegar have this action.

Anticatarrhal – herbs that will reduce the production mucus.

Antifungal – helps the body kill or inactivate fungi or fungal infections.

Antihaemorrhagic – a herb with astringent actions that can help be effective at stopping mild or moderate internal bleeding.

Antihistamine – a herb that will reduce the severity of allergic reactions.

Anti-inflammatory – any remedy that reduces inflammation in the body, although herbs tend to work more by aiding the inflammation to cleanse the area, rather than suppressing the inflammatory process.

Antilithic – a herb that can help break up or dissolve kidney or bladder stones.

Antimicrobial – a herb that will destroy or inhibit disease-causing bacteria.

Antimitotic – inhibits cell division.

Antiparasitic – having an action against parasites.

Antispasmodic – reducing spasm or tension particularly in areas of smooth muscle, such as gut walls, bronchial tubes, etc.

Antiviral – a herb that will suppress the growth of viruses.

Astringent – having a binding or contracting action on mucous membranes and tissue, usually because of the presence of tannins.

Auto-immune – an abnormal reaction of the body to its own cells, which the immune system attacks.

Bronchodilator – a herb that will help open up the airways.

Cystitis – inflammation of the bladder causing scalding pain when passing urine.

Demulcent – having the action of soothing and protecting membranes, notably in the gut, mouth, throat, urinary system, skin and wounds. Normally due to the mucilage content which has a characteristic 'slimy' consistency.

Depurative – a herb that has a blood-purifying or alterative action.

Diuretic – to provoke an increase in the flow of urine.

Electrolytes – the natural salts, e.g. sodium chloride, sodium bicarbonate, potassium chloride, that are present in solution in the body. Loss of electrolytes through sweating, for example, can cause dehydration and exhaustion.

Euthanasia – the painless killing of an animal suffering from an incurable disease or on welfare grounds.

Expectorant – having the action of encouraging the passage of mucus up the bronchials.

Febrifuge – herb that will reduce high temperature by increasing sweating and dilating blood vessels.

Hydroponic – grown in water.

Incontinence – bladder instability leading to loss of control over urination.

Laxative – promotes bowel movements.

MRSA – methicillin-resistant *Staphylococcus aureus*.

NSAID – non-steroidal anti-inflammatory.

Prophylactic – a herb that can be used to help strengthen the immune system, thereby assisting the body's defences against disease.

Refrigerant – a herb having a cooling action that will relieve fever and thirst.

Tranquilliser – a plant that will reduce excitability, without disturbing co-ordination or brain function.

Urethritis – inflammation of the urethra.

Vasodilator – an agent that causes widening of the blood vessels.

Vermicide – a substance that is poisonous to worms.

Vermifuge – worm expellant action on the intestine.

USEFUL ADDRESSES

Veteran Horse Society
Head Office and Rehabilitation Centre
Hendre Fawr Farm
St Dogmaels
Cardigan
North Pembrokeshire
SA43 3LZ
Tel: 0870 2426653
email: info@veteran-horse-society.co.uk
website: www.veteran-horse-society.co.uk

British Association of Equine Dental Technicians
Tel: 01827 284718
www.equinedentistry.org.uk.

British Association of Homeopathic Veterinary Surgeons
Chinham House
Stanford-in-the-Vale
Faringdon
Oxfordshire
SN7 8NQ
Tel: 01367 710324

Homeopathic Trust and Faculty of Homeopathy
Tel: 0207 566 7800

British Holistic Veterinary Medicine Association
Tel: 01273 725951

National Institute of Medical Herbalists (NIMH)
Elm House
54 Mary Arches Street
Exeter
Devon
EX4 3BA
Tel: 01392 426022
website: www.NIMH.org.uk

Tree of Remembrance Scheme
The International League for the
    Protection of Horses (ILPH)
Anne Colvin House
Snetterton
Norwich
Norfolk
NR16 2LR
Tel: 0870 3666913
email: Bevs@ilph.org

American Holistic Veterinary Medicines Association
website: www. AHVMA.org
A US organisation that supports holistic, complementary and alternative veterinary medicine, and natural healing for pets and animals.

Veterinary Botanical Medicines Assn
www.VBMA.org
An on-line resource for veterinary botanical medicine, veterinary herbal and phytomedicine, herbalism, herbology, and phytotherapy.

National Animal Supplement Council (NASC)
website: www.nasc.cc
A USA industry group (principally feed supplements manufacturers) dedicated to protecting and enhancing the health of companion animals and horses throughout the USA. Members of this group comply with an independently audited quality control standard similar to the European Universal Feed Assurance System (UFAS). (Hilton Herbs is a member of both the NASC and UFAS.)

HERBAL AND HOMEOPATHIC SUPPLIERS

Hilton Herbs
Downclose Farm
North Perrott
Somerset
TA18 7SH
Tel: 01460 270700
email: helpline@hiltonherbs.com
website: hiltonherbs.com

Ainsworths Homeopathic Chemists
38 New Cavendish Street
London
W1M 7LH
Tel: 01883 340332

Chamisa Ridge Inc,
3212 A, Richards Lane
Santa Fe
New Mexico 87505
USA
Tel: 1-505-438-4811
Fax: 1-505-438-8205
website: www.chamisaridge.com
This company is the USA distributor of Hilton Herbs products and offers an excellent selection of complementary healthcare products for animals.

RECOMMENDED READING

Complete Holistic Care and Healing for Horses, Mary Brennan – 2001, Kenilworth Press (Buckingham, UK) and Trafalgar Square Publishing (Vermont, USA)

Horses and Homeopathy – A Guide for Yard and Stable, Mark Elliot and Tony Pinkus, 1994, Ainsworths (London)

Bach Flower Remedies for Animals, Graham and Vlamis, 1999, Findhorn Press (Scotland)

Modern Horse Herbal, Hilary Self, 1996 (hardback) and 2004 (paperback), Kenilworth Press (Buckingham, UK)

Bach Flower Remedies for Horse and Rider, Martin Scott and Gail Mariani, Kenilworth Press (Buckingham, UK)

Threshold Picture Guides – Kenilworth Press (Buckingham, UK)

  No. 38 Massage for Horses, Mary Bromily (1996)

  No. 40 Aromatherapy for Horses, Caroline Ingraham (1997)

  No. 44 Homeopathy, Christopher Day (2000)

  No. 48 Caring for Older Horses and Ponies, Susan McBane (2004)

Herbal Handbook for Farm and Stable, Juliette de Bairacli Levy, 1988, Faber and Faber (London)

Wild Health, Cindy Engel, 2003 (paperback), Phoenix (Orion Books, London) and Houghton Mifflin Co. (USA)

Complementary Therapies for Horse and Rider, McBane and Davis, 2001, David and Charles (Newton Abbot, UK)

Beech, J., Garcia, M.C., 1985, 'Hormonal responses to TRH in healthy horses and horses with pituitary adenoma'. *American Journal of Veterinary Research* 46: 1841–1843

INDEX

Note: Page numbers in **bold** refer to illustrations in the text.

abscess, mouth 58
abscesses 76
ACTH (adrenocorticotrophin hormone) 33
adaptogens 87
age, records 10
ageing 8
alcohol 18
alfalfa 66
allergies 24–6, 60
   food 26
   respiratory 24–6, 60
   seasonal 25–6, 62
allicin 45, 62, 83
aloe vera 19, 74
Alternative Medicine Review 36
analgesics 29
aniseed 45, 61
anthelmintic herbs 82–4
anti-inflammatory herbs 29
antibiotics 38–9, 45
anticancer herbs 56–7, 65
anticatarrhal herbs 61
antihistamines 62
antilithics 71
antimicrobial herbs 62, 65, 67
antimitotic herbs 56–7
antiparasitic herbs 82–4
antiseptic herbs 62, 65, 67, 74–5
   urinary system 68, 69
antispasmodic herbs 40
antiviral herbs 63, 65
appetite, lack of 27–8, 45
Armstrong, Sue 51
arnica 31, 67, 76, 86
arthritis 29–32
Arthur **10**
artichoke 37, 45, 53, 80
ash, prickly 29, 30
aspen 71
aspirin 43
astringent herbs 61, 71, 74

aucubin 46, 61, 62, 72

Bach Flower remedies 21–2
   appetite loss 28
   arthritis 32
   competition 88
   Cushing's Disease 39
   digestive disorders 42
   euthanasia and bereavement 91–2
   eyes 48
   melanoma 57
   Rescue/Recovery 21, 42, 64, 78, 88
   respiratory problems 64
   urinary problems 71
   wounds 78
bacteria, gut 80–1
Badger 10
bandages 31, 86
bark, decoctions 17
barley 27
bedding 60, 87
bilberry fruit 29, 37–8, 46
birch 69
bitter herbs 28, 45, 53
bladder stones 71–2
bleeding 77
boiled grains 27
boneset 29, 62
bronchodilators 62
bruising 77
burdock 17, 30, 51, 53, 76
burial 90

calendula **19**, 44, 45, 49, 50, 55, 59, 63, 65, 70, 75, 78
   tinctures 56, 67
cancer 32
   see also melanoma
cayenne 30
celery seed 30

chamomile 25, 40–1, 45, 47, 59, 62, 69, 75
chaste tree 35–6, **37**
cherry plum 71
chimpanzees 83
cider vinegar 31
circulation, feet 48–9
circulatory stimulants 29
CITES (Convention on International Trade in Endangered Species) 16
clary sage 47
cleavers 12, 30, 31, 49, 50, 51, 55, 58
colic 40–2
collection of herbs 13–14
coltsfoot 61, 62
comfrey 31, 44, 61, 62, 75, **75**
commercial herbs 15–16
companions, loss of 91–2
competition, veteran horses 10, 85–8
compresses 20, 77
corn silk 70, 72
corns 48–9
couch grass 50–1, 55, 70, 72
coughs 59–64
crab apple 39, 57, 64, 71, 78
cramp bark 40, 45
creams 18, 77
cremation 90
Cushing's Disease 32–9, 57, 70
cystitis 70

dandelion 30, 41, 45, 51, 53, 69, **73**
death 89–92
decoctions 17
demulcents 70, 71, 72
depurative herbs 30
devil's claw 16, 29
dexamethasone suppression test 34

diet 79–80
  see also feeding
digestive disorders 40–5
digestive system 40, 80–1, 87
  see also worming
Ditton 6, **9**, 91–2
diuretics 69
domesticated horse 8–9
dopamine 35
dosages 11, 21, 22
drinking, encouraging 68, 86
Dryden, John 11
drying of herbs 14

echinacea 25, 38, 47, 50, **51**,
  55, 59, 75
elder 69
elderflower 47, 61, 62
elecampane 25, 50, 62, 84
electrolytes 86
elm 48
  slippery 20, 44, 45, 76
endangered plants 15–16
Engel, Cindy 83
Equine Event, UK 9
essential oils 17, 20, 31, 49, 86
  and digestion 45
  inhalation 20, 60–1
  massage 31, 86
eucalyptus 49, 60
euphrasia 48, 78
euthanasia 89, 91–2
expectorants 61
eye problems 37, 46–8
eyebaths 19, 26, 47
eyebright 26, 46, 47, 61

Fair Trade organisations 16
fatty acids, essential 38
febrifuge 62
feeding 27–8, 66, 79–80
  of herbs 16, 17
  pre- and probiotics 80–1
  rejection of herbs 12–13
  weight/appetite loss 27–8
fennel 45, 47

fenugreek 28, 65, 66, 75
feral horse 8
first aid 74–8
fish oils 38
'flu vaccines 51–2
food allergies 26
foot problems 48–9
fresh herbs
  collection 13–14
  dosages 21
fructo-oligosaccharides (FOS)
  80
fruits, feeding 79

garlic 25, 45, 49, 50, 58, 61,
  62, 80, 81, 83
gastric ulceration 42–4
gentian 28
ginger 29, 31
ginkgo 29, 46, **47**
glucocorticoids 33
goat's rue 38
golden rod 37, 70, 71
golden-seal 15–16, 50
gorse 39
gotu kola 41, 44, 45, 75, 76
gravel root 71
gums (horse's) 57–9, 66

Harman, Joyce 36
harvesting, of herbs 13–14
hawthorn 13, 29
haylage 24, 27
healing 74, 75
hedgerows 12
hemp oil 38
Holistic Veterinary Medicine
  Association 51
homeopathic remedies 22
  arthritis 32
  competition 87–9
  Cushing's disease 39
  digestive problems 42
  eye problems 48
  melanoma 57
  respiratory problems 26, 63

homeopathic remedies *cont.*
  rules for use 23
  sarcoids 65
  tooth problems 67
  vaccinations 52
  wounds 78
honey 78
hoof problems 48–9
horehound, white 62
hornbeam 39, 57
Hudson Bay 10
hydrangea, wild 72
hypericum (St John's wort) 29,
  56, 67, 78
hypericum and calendula
  tincture 67
hypothalamus 33
hyssop 61

immune system 49–52, 57
immunisations 51–2
impatiens 42
incontinence 70–1
infection 50
  sinuses 58, 67–8
  urinary 68–70
  wounds 77
inflammation
  bowel 44, 45
  urinary tract 70
  wounds 77
infusions 16–17
inhalers 20, 60–1
insulin resistance 38
insurance 85
International League for the
  Protection of Horses (ILPH)
  90

kidney disease 68, 69
kidney stones 71–2
kidney support 70

lameness 52–3
laminitis 32, 33, 38, 48
larch 48

lavender 31, 45
laxatives 41
legs, care of 31, 86
lemon balm 61
lime flowers 69
linseed 27, 66
liquorice 25, 41, 44, 45, 58, 61, 62, 70
liver 36–7, 51, 53–4
lovage 45
lymphatic herbs 30
lymphatic system 54–5

magnetic rugs and leg wraps **30**, 31, 86
marshmallow leaf 61, 62, 70, 72
marshmallow root 20, 43–4, 45, 62, 76
massage 31, 86
meadowsweet 29, 30, 43, 62, 69, 86
melanomas 56–7, 72
menthol 45
milk thistle **2**, 36–7, 51, 53–4, **54**, 81
mint 28, 45
moon blindness 48
mouth ulcers 57–9, 67
MRSA (methicillin-resistant *Staphylococcus aureus*) 62
MSM (methyl sulphonyl methane) 38, 49
mucilages 43–4, 62
mucous membranes 60
mucus 24–5, 60
mugwort 84
mullein 58, 61
muscle wastage 53, 59
myrrh 45, 49, 50, 58, 67

navicular 32
nettle 26, 29, 31, 62, 69
nose veil 26
nosebag inhaler 20, 60–1
nosodes 57

NSAIDs (non-steroidal anti-inflammatory drugs) 30, 38–9

oak 39
oats 80
oils
    essential, *see* essential oils
    feeding 79
    fish 38
    hemp 38
ointments 18, 77
olive 39, 88
onions 80
organic herbs 15

pain 77
parotid gland swelling 55
peppermint 45, 62
peppermint oil 31
pergolide 35
periodontal pocketing 66
phenylbutazone 30
photosensitive reactions 29
pituitary gland 33
plantain 25, 47, 50, 58, 61, **62**, 62, 72
plants
    collection 13–14
    endangered 15–16
    identification 93
pollens 25
potassium 69
poultices 19–20, 76
prebiotics 45, 80, 81
pregnancy 68, 83
preparations 16–20
probiotics 30, 42, 45, 80–1, 87

refrigerants 61
rejection, of herbs 12
respiratory problems 59–64
respiratory system 87
rheumatism, *see* arthritis
rhizomes 14

roots 14
rose hips 49
rosemary 30, 45, 46–7, 86
rosmarinicin 47
rugs, magnetic **30**, 31, 86

sage 58–9, 62, 67
St John's wort (hypericum) 29, 56, 67, 78
sarcoids 64–5, 72
scleranthus 39
seaweed 49, 55
self medication 83
Shakespeare, William 89
sheath, cleaning 72–3
silica 78
sinus infections 58, 67–8
sources of herbs
    commercial 15–16
    local 12–13
southernwood 84
soya beans 80
sprays
    skin/wounds 19, 74
    stables/horseboxes 60, 87
stable management
    at competitions 86
    respiratory problems 60
    winter 27
storage of herbs 14–15, 17
stress 27, 87
sugar beet 28, **66**, 86
sulphur 49
'superbugs' 62
swellings, glandular 55

tablets, administration 23
tack fitting 53
tansy 84
tea tree oil 49, 60
teeth
    care of 53, 65–6, **82**, 83
    problems 58, 66–8
thrush 49
thuja 52, 56–7
thujone 83, 84

thyme 25, 45, 50, 60, 61, 62, 84

thymol 84

tinctures 18, 21

topical applications 18, 31

trade, in herbs 15–16

travelling 87

Tree of Remembrance Scheme (ILPH) 90

turmeric 29

ulceration
  gastric 42–4
  mouth 57–9, 67
  skin 76
urinary antiseptics 68, 69
urinary problems 68–71
urinary stones/gravel 71–2

vaccinations 51–2
valerian 40, 41, 45
vasodilators 29
vegetables, feeding 79
veteran horse
  caring for 8–9
  record ages 10
  value of 9, 85–6
Veteran Horse Society (VHS) 10
vision 37, 46
vitamin C 57, 65, 75
vitamin E 75
Vitex agnus castus 35–6, 37

walnut 88
warming herbs 29–30
washes 19

water supply 79
weight loss 27–8
Wild Health (Engel) 83
willow 29, 31, 62
winter management 27
witch hazel 49, 56, 67, 74, 75, 86
withania 87
worming 81, 82–4
wormwood 45, 84
wounds 74–8

yarrow 29, 45, 53, 62, 69–70
yoghurt 81

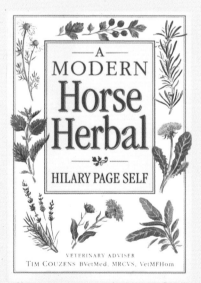

BY THE SAME AUTHOR

A MODERN Horse Herbal

HILARY PAGE SELF

VETERINARY ADVISER
TIM COUZENS BVetMed, MRCVS, VetMFHom

*Available from good bookshops and saddlers, or direct from
Kenilworth Press, Addington, Buckingham, MK18 2JR
tel: 01296 715101 or visit the website:*
www.kenilworthpress.co.uk
to order on-line